# Dy

A PRACTICAL GUIDE
FOR THE JOURNEY

# Dying

## A PRACTICAL GUIDE
## FOR THE JOURNEY

## Sue Wood and Peter Fox

DOUBLE
STOREY
a juta company

This edition published 2005 by Double Storey Books,
a division of Juta & Co. Ltd, Mercury Crescent,
Wetton, Cape Town

ISBN 1-77013-017-9

Page layout by Claudine Willatt-Bate
Cover design by Nic Jooste
Printing by Creda Communications, Epping, Cape Town

# Contents

# Dedication

To Catherine Mary – For all you taught us, and for your courage, dignity and determination. At times your circumstances tested those close to you to the limit and beyond. You were patient with us when we were overbearing with good intention. For direct honesty, humour and integrity in the acceptance of the most important journey of your life. Your spirit shines on. Thank you.

*Sue Wood*


To Gerda – Your death in 1983 in the face of the limitations of medicine and the aloneness of your suffering have been an instructive source of rich learning and insight for me. The courage, faith and spiritual questing of your life remain an inspiration.

*Peter Fox*

# Dear Reader

This book is about the realities of the terminal phase of illness.

Our intention is to help anyone who is dying. We discuss what we and others have found happening then – what you can expect, what others have found important to do, generally how to respond positively and practically to what you are likely to meet on this unfamiliar and perhaps hard road. The book is primarily to help you, your family and friends as you journey along together.

The book is also for anyone who will be involved in day-to-day care and nursing. We aim to help the lay carer to deal with the distressing difficulties and challenges and to enhance the dignity and comfort of all concerned. We address the professionals too, offering well-tested ideas on how to act in circumstances that are always difficult to handle, whatever one's training and experience.

The suggestions and observations are gleaned from our practical experience. Many of these insights are precious lessons that the dying teach the living. We have researched all the options mentioned and sought the critiques of medical personnel, aware that this area of medical and spiritual expertise is alive with varying opinions.

It is up to individual readers to choose what they find helpful in the text.

We hope that all who read this book will find some consolation and positive assistance at a difficult time. Both of us believe in life after death and also in God (Peter as a Christian) but we have addressed spiritual matters in a generalised way as all people are affected, whatever their belief or lack of belief.

*Sue Wood and Peter Fox*
Cape Town
February 2005

Death and I shall meet, and when He plunges
His sword into me, He shall find me fully awake.

*Dag Hammarskjöld*

# 1
# The voice of destiny: Getting the news

Death is the final stage of growth in this life. There is no total death – only the body dies. The self or spirit or whatever else you may wish to label it is eternal.

*Elisabeth Kübler-Ross*

The clay out of which God formed me was flung to the ground and shattered.

*Beverley Rycroft*

We are numb. Our brains blur out the information we have just received. We cannot even speak. We are seated in a clinic in front of the physician or community nurse, emotions in turmoil, doing battle with anxiety. In a brief moment the path of the future changes, forever. The confirmation of terminal illness is spelt out: 'There is nothing more we can do.' This has been a possibility since the original diagnosis and during the ordeal of the treatments. Hope for a miracle lies in tatters, leaving anger, bewilderment and despair in its place. This reality shocks, and elicits strong and mixed emotions. Remission is over. In some cases it had never begun.

How on earth do we prepare for our farewell? How do we leave behind all that has been precious and important to us? If we can find some answers here, then the life we have left can become a positive, hope-filled experience.

**First responses to the knock on our door**
What happens when we are confronted with the realities of the news? Fear may override our rational thinking. Reading the distressing symptoms that indicate significant changes in the body, we may grow afraid that we won't be able to control our normal functions. We could lose, or may have already lost, most of our hair. We experience weight loss of over ten kilograms. Our abdomen may distend and hang as if pregnant. We feel depressed, lost, embarrassed and humiliated. We will become dependent on others. We long for emotional, physical and spiritual support.

There may be different reactions. This is understandable, because although many people travel this road every day, they themselves vary. Here are some of their responses:
- fear
- hoping that it will just go away
- refusing to discuss the diagnosis with anyone

- promising to 'deal with it' after special religious holy days and holidays, birthdays, an anniversary, a vacation, or some other occasion
- feelings of failure, self-accusation, and guilt
- deep regret about lifestyle choices that could have been different
- anxiety about the sufficiency of finances.

But some choose to face their circumstance head on. This will ensure that the suffering is not triumphant, and does not take total power. It means summoning up as much courage as possible, from a place of emotional honesty and vulnerability. There is a lot to take in and process. You will need time and you will not want to be rushed.

Death is a perfectly natural part of the cycle of life – in all the realms of nature. While we know this intellectually, we find it difficult to accept emotionally. Is it our normal fear of the unknown that looms like a monster in the dark? Or it could be the old adage, We don't fear the unknown so much, but the loss of the known.

Perhaps because we exist individually, the extinguishing of this individuality is what we fear. There may be panic about unfulfilled longing in us. Eventually we might get to a realistic stage where we can talk about what matters to us and to those we love. Then we can begin to touch on practical issues that need our attention. Many of us are reluctant to investigate or consider certain issues. But these are unavoidable: we need to deal with them in order to ease the negotiation of and the journey into the unknown – what Shakespeare calls 'the undiscovered country from whose bourn no traveller returns'. If it is approached in fear, it is indeed a frightening path that looms ahead.

Denial at this stage is fierce: anger, fear, bitterness and disappointment become unwelcome companions. Sometimes just an overwhelming sadness and sense of isolation descends upon us. Skilled counselling for you and your partner or carer can help. But some people have great difficulty (especially at this stage) even considering this type of assistance, as it can often be seen as 'giving in to the inevitable' or, even worse, acceptance of the relentless approach of death. Feelings of failure are common, particularly in the area of faith in God or a higher purpose – whatever beliefs we follow. To those of us who trust in God, it can seem that He has abandoned us, left us to our own devices.

In the Western world, death is negatively perceived and so it is programmed out of our inner vision. There is a mental sign in front of us that shouts: 'Don't go there!' But this is the time for the ultimate questions: 'Who am I? Why am I here? What is and has been the purpose of my life?' Our physical life is running out on us, so our spiritual being comes to the fore, and we need to know where we are and what to do. If we have no roadmap for this exploration, we tend to get lost in a dark forest of speculation or wander on a desert plain if we are without any ideas on the subject.

We need to discover what brings us comfort, peace and hope, even in this seemingly hopeless situation, so that our passage through this crisis is manageable and positive. These matters are discussed in Chapters 5, 6 and 9 below, and dwelt on further in the Appendix.

## Sharing the situation

Life crises often have the capacity to provoke unexpected, puzzling and insensitive reactions from those around us. If we are dying, some of our anxiety is related to the probable loss of independence of movement and control over our bodily functions. It is here that acceptance of the immediate circumstances is most helpful. Once strain and resistance are absent, mental tension eases, opening the way for constructive planning; and muscular tension eases too, so the weakened body is relieved of stress and can function better as a result.

Joe,[1] a 40-year-old father with two children, said to Peter on the ward, 'How do I face my children? I can't hold them any more. They see their Dad weak and pathetic in this bed. I hate what is happening for them!' There are no trite answers to this statement, but we can ask: What resources lie within the person suffering? What support is there in the surrounding community? The list includes resources of real listening, relaxation and meditation, working with anger; and for Joe, finding a loving connection with his children, who will remember what their father wanted and hoped for them before he died. If Joe can access these resources, he can open up a different reality.

And for those of us in the caring circle, how do we respond when we know that someone we love is dying? Sometimes our first reaction is to blame: 'You must have done something wrong' or 'If only that check-up had been done earlier' or 'You have been tempting fate' or 'You should not have smoked as much as you did.'

Self-righteous remarks and attitudes just add to and compound strong feelings of guilt, despair and failure in the already suffering and fearful person. Appropriate responses could be: 'How do you feel your body speaks to you now?' or 'What resources are going to be important to you now?' Try to avoid expressing judgement, making evaluations and offering opinions. Simply try to express sadness, love and concern – for none of us knows what life has in store for us, and truly we must each say, 'There but for the grace of God go I.' The theologian Paul Tournier suggests that the prime duty of love is to *listen*.

For the dying person and the carers too: Try to steer clear of those who, for whatever reason, insensitively pass judgements on how and why things have turned out this way. People can tend towards harsh self-criticism, judgement, punishment, and inability to forgive the self.

Negative opinions like these mercilessly stoke the fires of guilt and worthlessness in us.

Here it is important to remember that the whole caring circle is involved: family and friends. We as carers encircle the ill person and are deeply affected by what happens in the household. The illness disrupts our lives on a daily basis, and so we are very vulnerable in the face of criticism.

**Guidelines after the death verdict**

Here are some guidelines for you and any companion as you leave the consulting room, the words ringing in your ears. We have taken these suggestions from the lips of the dying – those who have shared their truths with us. They are not offered in any particular order.

**Try to live in the present**, moment to moment. Live each day dealing with the day as it is, good or bad. Dwell neither in the past nor in the future. Treasure quality times all the time. This requires mental discipline and practice, because human beings are so conditioned and manipulated not to be in the present. The power of the present moment can be appreciated for the important reality it is. The moment will pass, but its imprint will have been made.

**Pace and clear your life.** Take one step at a time and keep things as simple as possible. Determine what is truly important, focus on it, and discard the rest. Shed unnecessary baggage.

**Deal with unfinished business.** It can be as toxic as a fatal disease, and often causes prolonged suffering as we cling desperately to the last threads of physical existence. This brings untold distress to the loved ones and the ill person in particular. Dealing with unfinished business – wherever possible – eases the path to death without distractions.

**Get real.** Talking about what really matters is difficult enough while we are in good health, let alone facing the end of our life as we know it. Total honesty with the self helps in this tricky task.

**Clear blocked relationships.** Do not expect full co-operation from those with whom you have had disagreement or where there is bad blood. Clear the situation, taking responsibility for your own action and reactions, and set yourself and the other parties free. Where resolution simply cannot be achieved, you can at least agree to disagree without resentment.

**Avoid recrimination.** Accept the deep regrets of rifts in relationships that remain unresolved, where important things will be left unsaid.

**Forgive yourself and others.** The gift of forgiveness, for the self and others, makes the soul lighter at a time when the body is so heavy and tired.

**Find a place for laughter.** A good sense of humour, an ability to see the funny side in the tragedy, is not only healthy but also refreshing.

**Seek assistance.** If necessary, seek the expertise of competent counsellors and social workers. Get yourself a spiritual counsellor. If you find that the one of your choice is not able to assist you, find another. Confidentiality is vital, as it is your very soul that is being laid bare.

**Create a support circle.** It's never too late to find a small group of friends or family with whom you are able to develop an honest and trusting relationship. They will help you on this, the most important journey of your life.

**Find a safe place of refuge.** This could be your church, synagogue, mosque, Sufi temple, retreat, or another place that is special for you. Find the one that suits you, and seek ways to use the strengths that are nurtured in this place of peace and quiet.

**Express your feelings** to whoever accompanied you to the doctor. Sudden exposure to shattering, life-changing news is terrifying even though the possibility has existed since initial diagnosis. Before attempting the arduous task of trying to break the news to others, try to cry out or express immediate reactions together with your companion to help release the torrent of feeling within. Take *time* for this; do not be rushed. (We address this early situation in greater detail in the next chapter.)

**Contact your health practitioner.** Where possible, make an appointment with a reputable homeopath, doctor or other practitioner of your choice to assist you with medication for shock, depression and trauma as First Aid helps. Rescue Remedy (see Chapter 8) is invaluable here for all concerned.

You may well have registered with a good general practitioner or with a day hospital if your diagnosis was of cancer or HIV/Aids. If you are not registered with either at this time of advanced illness, we recommend that you do so as soon as possible. If you do decide to register, first check if your health care practitioner is prepared to help by visiting you at home. Similarly, ask what the day hospital can offer by way of home visits and support. Some services may only apply in cities, not the smaller towns and rural areas.

The extra support is invaluable, as regular visits from those with medical expertise do help you, the sufferer. If registered with Hospice, you can leave the rest to them: this area is well supervised by the Hospice medical team. It is important to have your own general practitioner even if Hospice is part of your support system.

**Approach your local Hospice for information.** If you have Hospice in your area, register with them to keep your options open; your needs will change with the advancing stages of your condition. Hospice offers invaluable services in counselling and support for you and, equally importantly, for your family and carers.

The purpose of Hospice is to promote the dignity of life, to manage and alleviate pain, and to give some measure of control back to the patient. An early referral enables maximum benefit to be drawn from all the services that Hospice offers in their interdisciplinary teamwork and facilitation of family needs. Please note: Not every Hospice is able to provide all the services we mention in this book, and some geographical areas may currently be out of Hospice reach.

Some people do not approach Hospice for help because they perceive Hospice as a symbol of demise, 'the end'. Denial and avoidance often cause us to resist and hold back until all other options are exhausted.

It is most important to understand that denial may well be the only defence mechanism that the patient has at this time. Compassionate, skilful counselling is needed here, as one cannot simply break the denial without other mechanisms in place.

By the same token, it is very helpful if people try to address this resistant mindset early on, to equip all parties concerned with the skills to transform the reality of approaching death from one of fear and denial to one of peace and gentle transition.

**Understand that you are entering a process.** This process may involve treatments. Even a patient close to death may well benefit, for example, from a single fraction of radiotherapy to excruciatingly painful ribs in the case of breast cancer.

The process may also involve leaving the hospital and going home to die. The change from receiving anticancer care to mainly home-based symptomatic control is a transition rather than a point. Those around you may need to lead you gently into the next phase – your ability to accept new steps in the process is very important for your emotional wellbeing.

Try to remember that now is not the time for misplaced heroism and pride. Pride and stubbornness are expensive attitudes when you need to keep your dignity and integrity, and above all comfort and peace for your ailing body. Throughout the process, everyone needs to focus on the quality of life, care, love and help.

**Move towards acceptance.** There is a story of someone who was in meditation. A friend approached and said, 'How can you sit there when there is so much pain and suffering in the world?' The meditator picked up a drinking glass. 'You see this glass? I hold it up and it reflects the light. I pour a little water into it, tap it, and it makes music. But the wind or my elbow could easily knock it off the shelf and shatter it. So I presume that the glass is already broken, and I enjoy the moment of it.' As we contemplate the most uncomfortable reality of our impending death, when inside we are shouting No, it is still possible to live in the moment and even enjoy it.

**Note**

1  Patients referred to by their first name only have been given pseudonyms to protect their anonymity.

# 2
# Breaking the news, and after

Midway in this life we're bound upon,
I awoke to find myself in a dark wood
Where the road was wholly lost and gone.

*Dante Alighieri, The Inferno*

## Giving the news: For the professional

Telling someone they are terminally ill is a hard task, and can be unpleasant. The temptation is to rush it, and then the news often gets blurted out in a manner that comes across as cruel and unfeeling. Another negative way is to be vague. Here, the health care professional can simply fudge the issue. The patient is left trying to work out what is being said.

How you give the news will affect the way the patient manages afterwards. A clumsy, impatient, insensitive manner will create problems. The patient's anger and resentment may be more likely to carry on into the future of living with the illness.

Since there is no easy way to break bad news, or to

hear it spoken, at least ensure that you are in a place of complete privacy, with no distractions or interruptions possible. Consult with others if necessary to judge if the patient should bring a close relative or friend when they come to hear the news. This may not be everyone's choice, but could be very helpful.

Share the news as early as possible, don't hold on to it. It is only fair that the information should go to the patient at once, since it is their life and death you are talking about and they should be given reasonable time to adapt to the life-shifts involved.

Frequently, when you give a serious diagnosis, it is not correctly heard the first time; many patients experience a 'blank-out'. It is crucial to realise that when people take in bad news they are having to adjust to information that changes their life. From the moment they hear the news, there is the way they lived before and the way they will live now. Perhaps you need to repeat it. Do so in a sensitive and open way.

At this point fear and anxiety can magnify the threat and plunge the hearer into hopelessness. Since further along the patient's course to death there are sometimes other steps to negotiate, explain one thing at a time. Speak slowly and simply, not using too many words. Though the patient might not hear your words, she or he will be sensitive to your tone and your body language. Be aware of how these are coming across.

Some patients may hear you say: 'There is nothing more we can do for you. What about a referral to Hospice?' They may misinterpret the words to mean that nobody can do anything more about the illness. To many, the mere mention of Hospice means nothing but dying. This causes confusion and fear in their mind. For them it implies that people at Hospice will now become the only role players in their life.

An experienced social worker at Hospice suggests making the referral in this way: 'We have come to the end of what I have been doing for treatment. In spite of all our efforts, your condition is no longer responding. We need to look realistically at the options you have now. There is another organisation that can assist us with the whole process. They should be able to help us as we go on working together.' This more honest approach caters for the patient's vulnerable state by emphasising that you are not rejecting their case at all but will continue with it.

It is helpful to try dealing early on with what the person feels and to offer appropriate openings such as: 'You must have many questions, there must be issues you want me to go over with you.' 'What is surfacing in your mind right now?' 'Are you just numb?' 'This must be very difficult to take in at the moment.' Ask questions until the patient has grasped the implications. Has what you have been saying been clearly understood? It is important to get full details about what is being experienced, what is

Here is Samantha's eloquent story of how she finally got the clear news of her impending death:

My lungs had been damaged for a long time. Suddenly I could not breathe unassisted, and collapsed. I was rushed to hospital in cardiac distress. I am an intelligent woman and knew deep down that this would probably be the end – but would not admit it then. I still had so much to do. My sons live overseas and I needed to visit them. I had also cancelled my trip to Egypt the month before because I could not breathe and felt awful. In truth I was simply too weak to travel. So there I was, lying in hospital. MRI scan, X-rays, blood tests and all those nasty invasions were revealing news that I could not persuade anyone to tell me. I knew this must be bad. The long silences. The raising of eyebrows by the attending doctor on examining my body or the contents of my file made me suspicious. I studied his body language and watched his facial expressions closely for some hint.

I became anxious, tense and angry. This made my breathing much more difficult. I confronted the doctor on the fourth day. 'I have to know what's happening to me. Please tell me honestly. I have to visit my sons overseas soon.

Can I travel by plane? I also live alone and must make plans for my care. If I am dying I have to tell my sons.' He shuffled the papers around, closed my file and shook his head. As he walked away from my bed he said: 'You won't be travelling anywhere for the time being.' And left.

It was then I knew and yet did not know. I simply had to find someone to tell me if I was really going to die. I cried in frustration. Everyone seemed to avoid meaningful conversation with me.

Out of the blue an hour or two later, an old friend arrived at my bedside. As I blurted out my sorry tale, tears pouring unchecked down my cheeks, she held my hand and listened quietly. When I was calm she suggested that I consult with her husband's nephew for a second opinion. He is a general practitioner. She kindly arranged for him to see me, after he had studied my case and consulted with the attending doctor.

I checked out of the hospital with a bottle of oxygen as my companion. He came – and spent three hours with me at my home privately. Bless him – he told me the truth. He heard my concerns and fears. With his help I can make plans for my care. I am so relieved. He spoke frankly but kindly. I am dying – I have a little time left, but at least I know what to do with it.[1]

not comprehended, and what the patient needs to know. For that, you need to communicate very clearly.

When patients surface from hearing the news, questions are likely to form in their minds: What symptoms can be expected? What, if any, treatments are available? What is the usual life expectancy for such a diagnosis? What about a second opinion? Provided that the patients' trust has been preserved and they know you are not forsaking them, medical knowledge can be given that will alleviate unnecessary anxiety and fear.

The dying frequently cannot cope with the emotional needs of those around them. Medical staff should be alert to these patients' wishes: respect for their needs is non-negotiable, and the same goes for their primary partner and carer. All visitors should do likewise: when visiting times are restricted, accept this well-meant boundary with generosity and understanding. To criticise having your visit refused will not help the carer; you will just be making life more difficult than it already is for those who are doing the best they can.

### Family rights and coordination
When the terminally ill person is a child and has biological parents who will not speak to each other under any circumstances, it may be helpful to ask them each to nominate a trusted representative to attend when you tell the young patient what is happening. They can bring

the questions that the parents want to ask, to be discussed in a round-table style. You need to set firm boundaries: you cannot become embroiled in the family politics. On the other hand, you can help facilitate a sensitive family discussion. Your main focus is to act in the interests of the patient, in consultation with the *primary* next of kin.

With adult patients, legally the primary next of kin is the current spouse. That person therefore comes before any children or the parents of either partner, and should be consulted first and on their own. If there is no spouse or other partner, then the person appointed by the patient as next of kin is respected as such – even if that person has no legal standing.

If it is clear that unresolved disagreements and ill feelings are going to predominate among those close to the patient, the only reasonable line you can take is to suggest they choose a spokesperson they can rely on. Call in bereavement counsellors, social workers, religious leaders or any other experienced people who are skilled in managing conflict resolution *positively*.

## Giving the news: For the dying and their circle

There comes a time when relatives and friends are puzzled about the health status of the patient and start to ask questions. If those in the know hide the truth in any way – by secrecy or nondisclosure of any kind – this only increases the isolation and inner anguish of the patient. This is not a time for anyone to be heroic, stoic, or sheltered from the facts.

Common-law partners in South Africa who live unwed as man and wife are not accepted as primary next of kin even if there is a contract between them. At the time of writing, this matter and the status of same-sex partners are being debated in the Constitutional Court and are *sub judice*. Where families have an agenda – for instance, an aversion to the current partner – the partner in a common-law relationship is thus at risk of being excluded legally by the primary next of kin from even being able to be with their loved one who is dying.

This is a volatile area that can explode into division, jealousy, bitterness and anger. In spite of all the feelings and legalities, remember the one who is dying. Their wishes need to be respected. The law is not compassionate, but people can be – we are capable of caring in abundance. We may be sorely tested when facing the death of a loved one. Counsellors skilled in conflict resolution can help here. A generosity of spirit in this truly prickly circumstance is vital for a peaceful transition for the seriously ill person, and for those who live on afterwards.

Sometimes family members try to collude with the doctors: 'Let's not tell her that she is dying.' This causes pain and humiliation. The truth will come out eventually anyway, and it will be all the worse when the patient discovers that others knew and withheld the information. A far better way is for the family to seek a counsellor who can help the one who is dying to live with the illness, to explore feelings and face fear in a way that grounds everyone in reality. Social workers with palliative care experience, or counsellors specialising in the areas of loss and grief, can assist both patients and their families.

We encourage you to ask questions of the doctors and carers. This helps them to communicate more detail. Their answers may not always be adequate – but 'I don't know' is often more honest and no less knowledgeable than answers that attempt to field every question.

Just as stifling the questions poses a problem for the doctor and carers, so the persistent questioner creates difficulty. When people are stressed and in anguish it is not easy to find the balance, but we should all try.

When Jane was dying in our care at the Hospice, she asked her husband not to tell their children. This caused the children severe distress and made them feel insecure. Sometimes the ill person instructs the primary next of kin not to divulge anything that could cause anxiety for the children and family. This complex situation can create a burden for the partner. Here it may be helpful for the partner to confide in a family doctor or spiritual counsellor. For Jane, we urged that she should do whatever would help her children treasure, value and remember her with gratitude. This required courage and inner strength on Jane's behalf.

When family members are shut out, they are likely to feel anger, guilt, shock and disbelief when the person dies. There are so many unanswered questions. Relatives out of town may experience deep regret or resentment at not having had the chance to visit the dying person in time.

**Circles of complication**
Around the dying there is often a circle of complicated relationships. How do we break the news when there is divorce, subsequent remarriage and step-families? What is the sensitivity and response needed when single-parent families confront the dying of a child or parent? Often the grandparents have to take on the responsibility.

A crisis can intensify the feelings of ambiguity that people hold for each other. Some marriages find themselves on the rocks. Spouses divorce; their children usually remain in their mother's care, with the father having visiting rights.[2] Second and even third marriages take place, bringing in the new spouse and their children.

What about the 'wicked' stepmother or stepfather? Often there are residual negative feelings between the ex-spouses which can affect the children. The children too can feel resentment and unhappiness and – as children do – behave badly and even cruelly as a result of their own pain. They might display a flagrant dislike of the step-parent, for example. Some families are plagued with favouritism – certain children are preferred, others excluded.

All of this breeds conflict, strong ill feelings, and anti-social behaviour and habits. Result: the inevitable break-down of loving, caring relationships and an increase of pain at all levels.

Provocation and coaching of children to relay messages of spite and malice by the ex-spouse are obviously unkind, and devastating to the child's perception of the parent to whom the malice is directed. Jealousy, jockeying for position, and manipulative, angry and resentful behaviour are a minefield even in physically healthy families, affecting adults and children alike. How much more so when someone is dying and everyone is under strain.

**Family manners**
Sharing the knowledge of terminal illness with parents, a spouse or children is essential but has its hazards. Whatever the circumstances, there is no useful place for personal agendas, pride, selfishness and negativity around the bedside of a dying person. Insecurity, hidden resentments, lack of forgiveness, regrets, and dispute or concerns about materialistic interest complicate matters. Displays of uncharacteristically selfish and self-centred

attitudes and behaviour can leave others in the family astonished and angry. Insensitive requests and discussion of the will can anger or hurt the dying person. These are the things that will fragment the family unity.

It is vital to contain the circumstances so that anger, shock, and any past conflict or other unfinished business do not snap the fragile threads that hold the family together and destroy the social fabric that exists. This is a tense time when conflict can flare up in people's own emotions and in their dealings with each other. Everyone in the family needs to take special care to behave well and keep focusing on the support and care of the one who is dying.

There is no set formula. People, professional or otherwise, each have their own emotional and intellectual reactions and coping mechanisms. Objective awareness, emotional honesty and mature decisions will help ease this difficult passage for all concerned.

**What do we say?**
Evasions or trite advice to the patient simply block the process of living with dying. These comments are all too familiar: Don't give up. You'll get over it. Everything changes with time. It could be worse, you know. You've had a good innings. We all have to die sometime. Every dark cloud has a silver lining. Be strong. Count your blessings. You must have done something wrong.

Carers have to accept the situation bravely and should not dispense with honesty in an effort to cheer up the ill person. They will only cause confusion if they say things like 'Don't be silly, of course you are going to get well'. Instead, encourage the patient to express the current experience and particularly feelings, by broaching the subject on these lines:

- I have no way of imagining or understanding what you are feeling. Please help me to understand.
- Have you gained anything in the experience of your illness? – things you have received that you didn't notice before, or things that you now see differently?
- Is there something inside you that you think might eventually comfort or console you?
- What is the strongest negative emotion you feel? – anger, fear, disappointment, rejection, or what?
- I can see your distress; what can I do to help? What is the best way I can be with you?

## Permission to let go

Fighting the disease process by stoically dealing with pain can add considerable stress to the overall mental, emotional and physical condition of people near death. Your permission to let go of the fight can help the dying one. Degeneration has taken its toll, the physical reserves are depleted or gone. If the carers and family accept this, everyone together can experience a new space of honesty and contentment of heart.

Carers have to search their own hearts. Do they want their loved one to keep living for their own emotional needs? Do they fear living without the person?

There is a time to let go. Part of the huge challenge for the patient is to know when this time has come. It is crucial not to make the person feel guilty for their shift in attitude. Their concerns then move to another horizon and are no longer about physical survival.

## Notes

1 As told to Sue.
2 The South African court, as upper guardian of children, considers a mother the best custodial parent unless this is proved otherwise. This is the norm in most countries.

# 3
# How on earth are we going to pay for this?

When my husband fell ill, we had our savings.
He is dead now and I am deep in debt.

*A patient's wife*

## Financial strains

It is a hard decision to face leaving work permanently because of ill health. As the illness progresses and the body becomes frail and exhausted, however, even part-time work becomes impossible.

The situation can be traumatic, whether it means medical boarding, resignation, or giving up a business. The family is faced with one income less, just when the prohibitively expensive treatments (particularly at private institutions) have cut deep into the spare income and savings, or perhaps exhausted them already. The shortfalls on medical aids can often result in debts, and so do exclusion clauses of medical insurance policies, and loss of income through taking time off from work.

Bonds may have to be extended and loans negotiated. Banks, usually so keen to lend money, turn down applications because the remaining income earner does not earn enough to cover the interest repayments. Professional home nursing may be needed, which means another bill to pay. Funeral costs will also have to be met when the person has died. All this makes an already distressing time intolerable: the family struggles to make ends meet while dealing with imminent death, and the dying person has the extra worry too.

### Sources of income

Some financial support could be available in the form of **state grants**. People may qualify for benefits such as an old age pension, a disability grant, or a grant-in-aid for someone who is a carer. The amounts are small – in 2004 the old age pension and disability grant were just R740 a month, while the grant-in-aid was only R160 – but many people in South Africa, often whole families, depend on them for their survival. Apply through the Department of Social Welfare, who will be able to tell you if you fit the criteria.

You may also be entitled to money from the **Unemployment Insurance Fund (UIF)** when you become too ill to continue working.[1] You must be a contributor to the UIF – this does not apply if you are self-employed, for instance. Make an appointment for an interview at your local Department of Labour, and take your documents with you.[2] (If you are too ill to travel, a family member can apply in your place, on proof of identification.) Ask what provision may be made for your dependants, if any. Discuss how you will be paid if you don't have a bank account and are too ill to collect your payments in person. UIF payments can take six to eight weeks to start after you have been assessed, so begin the process as soon as you leave your job.

To avoid potential financial problems, it is wise to create a **reserve account** for the next of kin to manage. This will allow funds to be accessible should the dying person become incapacitated. On death all other financial accounts will be frozen. The funds will then pass into the hands of the executor along with all other assets. The executor may only pay out a portion of the money available before the estate is wound up.

For those with **insurance policies** that have not been ceded to them directly, the proceeds will be paid into the estate. In that case, financial problems may continue long after death has occurred, as the winding up of the estate can take more than six months. There is some relief when insurance policies have been ceded to family members, however, because the proceeds are paid out to those beneficiaries within weeks of the death.

## Planning as a family

Whatever your circumstances, concerns about money are likely to be one of the most debilitating and stressful aspects of someone dying in your family. We urge you to explore your options at once. Then at least you will know you have done your best, and the family can set the subject aside as far as possible, turning their full attention to nonmaterial things.

If the prognosis is one to six months left of life, it is often wise for the partner to try spending as much time at home as possible. Depending on the attitude of the place of employment, plans for extended leave may be arranged. Some employers are generous and understanding, and will grant leave. Self-employment is different, of course, but some people have insurance cover for loss of income, which helps to ease the distress.

## Hospital options

Once you have the diagnosis of cancer or any other life-threatening disease, it is wise to ask firmly what options are available for treatment. You will need to learn what the projected costs of private treatment are likely to be, along with medical aid shortfalls and exclusions in your medical aid and medical insurance policies.

So often the emotional shock and fear at initial diagnosis blinds us. We don't ask these pertinent questions before choosing the route of treatment. There is no need to make a decision right there and then in the doctor's rooms. The ill person needs time to let the information sink in. Thirty-six hours' digestion and thinking time are not going to make any difference. Get all the hospital information you can. Consult with people who know and have experience in this area. Finally you, the patient, should choose what you feel at peace with.

Most patients if they have the means would normally choose private care rather than put up with the disadvantages of state hospitals. These include crowded waiting rooms, long waiting times, not seeing the same senior doctor on every visit, certain drugs not being available, and having to join waiting lists for some therapies. But find out what these places have to offer and what the costs will be, *despite the drawbacks*.

In many cases, state hospitals are worth considering. Currently there is an increase in the number of patients turning to government institutions after having started with private treatment because they cannot sustain the crippling cost. Most medical aids pay at the scheduled rate, which is much lower than the fees in private institutions. In addition, medical aids are changing their policies all the time. Nobody can guarantee what they will elect to pay in the future.

By choosing private care and then short-changing on various treatments because of the cost involved, some people unfortunately miss out on treatment options that they could have had very cheaply in a state hospital.

Another positive choice could be to visit the state hospital for initial confirmation of diagnosis, and consult with a combined panel for results and prognosis. At that stage you can decide whether to follow the public or private route, rather than rushing on with one option and then being forced to change when funds are no longer available. It can be counterproductive to get well known by one doctor and then be forced to change systems in the middle of treatment.

At the time of writing, the initiative of PPPs (public–private partnership hospitals) is slowly being implemented. Readers can explore the idea further by contacting their local hospitals for information. We include a useful website on public and private hospitals in the Contacts section at the end of this book.

If your financial position is already precarious, with substantial debts on which monthly repayments are made, a state hospital may well be the only option for continuing courses of treatment such as chemotherapy or radiotherapy. Prior to making a final choice, find out exactly what the medical aid will and won't cover. Always read the small print and check the exclusion clauses – benefits are frequently limited. Contact a person in a managerial position first and ask them to delegate an appropriate person to handle your case. Always note the name. It is wise to get written confirmation from the medical aid before committing yourself financially.

**Home care**

This is not so much an option these days as a reality once people are beyond the stage of treatment programmes and the illness is becoming terminal. As frailty increases, so does the need for nursing. Several choices are available. They are determined by the cost, your financial circumstances, and most of all by these very important factors:

- Does the dying person want to live and die at home?
- Can the carer and the family participate fully in the frail-care nursing and care? Family members can work well on a roster system with back-up from Hospice. There are some procedures that the lay person cannot cope with, either emotionally or simply because they do not 'have the stomach for it'. In that case, daily visits for tasks such as changing dressings of suppurating tumours by specialised staff can be provided by Hospice or nurses from nursing agencies. Sometimes Hospice can recommend registered nurses in private practice who specialise in home visits for changing dressings.
- Can you afford the day or night nurses provided by nursing agencies for part or all of the time?

St John Ambulance provides a training programme for home-care and frail-care skills at a reasonable cost. If there is a St John branch in your area, it's worth doing the course. Your domestic worker, if you have one, may also wish to do the training. Other people who have done the course already should be available if you need extra help. Contact your local St John Ambulance for more information.

The programme of care for your loved one can be well organised. It will have to have flexibility, as needs change.

**Hospice services**
Financial stress erodes the body and mind. It can result in ill health for the partner and children, and can cause severe family argument and disruption. This is one of the many reasons why it is invaluable to contact Hospice as soon as a life-threatening illness is diagnosed. Social workers come to the aid of the family. They facilitate the psycho-social support needed.

Counselling, nursing and equipment are supplied, frequently at little or no cost, depending on the financial position of the applicants. Hospice also offers support and home visits by specialised nursing sisters at nominal rates, charged in accordance with the financial position of the patient.

Admission to Hospice wards is arranged for rest and respite (for the patient and to give the family a break) for a specified time, for symptom and pain control, and for the last days of life. If there is no in-Hospice facility in your area, you may have to consider using state or private hospitals for these purposes instead.

Many of those reading this book are currently in good health. We hope our suggestions will equip you for the day when you or someone close to you is faced with terminal illness.

## Notes

1 UIF officers recommend that in the case of leaving work because of terminal illness, one does not resign but negotiates with the employer to be medically boarded.

2 Items you will need to take are: your ID book, a letter from your specialist, doctor (or otherwise your GP), your medical reports from oncologists, your last six months' original pay slips or certified copies of them, your UIF card filled in by your employer showing date of termination of employment, and a letter from your employer stating the terms of medical boarding and giving the reasons.

# 4
# The first days

The world is upside down
foreign, uncertain, changed for ever
an ending and a new beginning.

*Sue Wood and Peter Fox*

## Assembling the team, and caring for the living

The news that someone in the family is dying is like a stone thrown into a pond. The ripples begin. The visitors arrive. Routines are reshuffled. The family moves into a new space. These first days ask for creative responses, flexibility, boundaries and a new routine.

The dying person, if conscious, must be consulted and their decisions respected. The suggestions in this chapter are made in the full knowledge of just how painful and distressing the circumstances are for all concerned.

Teamwork is vital to the smooth flow of caring for the dying. Partners of ill people tend to overextend themselves for fear of being absent when they die. Don't take on too much yourself. We suggest you include family members in the daily chores. Allocate and delegate so that the household runs smoothly.

The first weeks can be a time of family solidarity and strengthening of connection – a time for family conferences. Ask those close to the dying person which tasks they would like to undertake and be able to perform. There are many routine jobs to do, such as producing regular meals. This is a time of new learning, understanding, compassion and acceptance of limitations. Personalities differ and some are better equipped to deal with certain tasks.

The main focus has to be on the dying person, but significant others in the family circle must also be noticed and cared for. Some spouses or partners are challenged in ways that stress them out. They need support themselves, and appreciation too.

We suggest that you pay special attention to any children in the home. Perhaps they could be given the first choice of tasks so they do not feel left out. Where much attention is given to the frail person, it is so easy to overlook the children's suffering. Children can sometimes feel responsible for causing the illness because that is how they tend to respond, and the situation is scary for them. Children see their parent, who is abandoning them (in their eyes) because of a disease against which all seem powerless, being brought gifts of flowers – being rewarded. This can hurt deeply, so offer them hugs and physical touch, affirming love and care.

Draw on all the circles of support. Lifts, shopping and general running around are good chores for willing friends. When help is offered, be clear what your requirements are and accept offers if appropriate.

People are generous and extremely kind, even more so under these circumstances. Small, considerate, helpful gestures will touch you. Try to acknowledge these whenever they occur.

Family members may resent the 'intrusion' of the many visitors – some of whom provide essential nursing and other services. It is true that family privacy can be compromised, but to some extent this may be a necessary fact that the family must try to accept. When resentment arises it needs to be aired and maybe a new path negotiated.

**Relaying the news**
'There goes the phone again. Somebody please answer it.' Phone calls and visiting can drain the primary carer or partner. Continuous repeated reporting on conditions and state of mind gets exhausting. One way to ease the load is by leaving a message on the telephone, as Sue did.

It saved my sanity recently, when my husband had open-heart surgery. I left an updated message on my answering machine twice a day, giving news of his condition. I did the same on voice-mail, on my cell phone. My husband's children, two of whom live overseas, could access updated information about their dad at all hours of the day or night while I was incommunicado.

I was saved having to repeat the news each time to many caring and concerned people, particularly when he contracted pneumonia in ICU. Exhaustion was my bugbear, so this simple tool allowed me space.

If you have access to the Internet, e-mail one message that can be sent to numerous addresses with a click of the mouse. A cell phone is also invaluable. It gives you full mobility, and you can keep in close touch by pressing a button. Incoming calls can be picked up, messages retrieved at a more convenient time, and the call returned.

Why not arrange for a few people to pass on updated reports on their lists of people? This go-between system works well.

While queries from well-meaning and deeply concerned people arise out of kindness, they can become a real intrusion. This is the time for clear boundaries. Map out priorities in consultation with your loved one; these would include who they wish to see (or not see), and when, and what business or other interests they want to attend to. Teamwork from all members of the household can come into play here so that these queries are answered graciously.

Tell family, friends and colleagues that they must phone before they visit. The frail person may suddenly have a bout of exhaustion or nausea, or may just feel unwell that day. The most important priority is the condition and choice of the one concerned.

## Bedside manners for visitors

Members of the wider family, children from previous marriages, very dear and close friends all want to see and spend time with their loved one. This can create stress for the dying person and also for the primary next of kin or partner, who frequently is the major carer.

If you are a visitor, offer assistance by providing simple meals for the family. Hearty soups, pasta dishes and fresh bread, along with salads or baskets of fruit, are always very welcome. Check what foods suit their allergies or dietary exclusion. Let the family be specific in their requests. Mark containers and dishes with your name. Clear communication of this kind just simplifies life for everyone.

The frailty of human nature means that there will be selfish displays as someone asserts their need to spend as much time as possible with the dying person. This calls for a firm, compassionate intervention by whoever is orchestrating the visits, as the dying person may often not be able to cope with the emotional needs of those around them. Respect for the dying person's needs and those of the primary partner or carer must come first.

As a visitor, accept that your visits may be restricted. It is not helpful to criticise the family if they limit when you may come. Are you being selfish? If so, shift your attitude. If there is an urgent, very real need to visit, then negotiate the circumstances sensitively.

Focus on the needs of your loved one who is dying. When visiting, try not to be self-focused. You are at the disposal of the dying person. Honesty, humility and sensitivity are helpful here.

Keep ever mindful of the need for tranquillity. Speak gently and quietly as you share your news during a visit. Sometimes saying very little – just sitting quietly holding hands – is much more beneficial than chatty conversation, which is normally exhausting. We suggest you stay away from life's dramas.

What matters is quality of life and contact, not the length of your contact, for whatever time is left. Don't overstay your welcome. Instead, keep visits short, with a keen eye on visible symptoms of exhaustion.

**Keeping the dying in mind**
The dying person is likely to have totally different priorities from those who are not facing imminent death.

Having a new focus does not mean that someone near death is losing their mind. On the contrary, the shift is usually a sign of alertness as people respond to the realities of dying.

Many make the harmful error of assuming that the ill person has become mentally infirm and isn't capable of making decisions. This is most often the source of frustration, tension and argument. Always discuss everything with your loved one, allowing them to make their own choices and decisions as far as they can. Where a decision is clearly inappropriate, discuss it again and offer constructive options.

The dying do not look for pity or sympathy, but they do need peace. Create a harmonious atmosphere. They are in distress, so straining them further with subjects about which they can do nothing is not only insensitive but cruel.

There will be days when everyone around will be subjected to a depressed, argumentative, demanding and grumpy patient. The team of carers and close family will also have days when it just gets too much, and they will also have feelings of frustration and irritation born of exhaustion and distress.

This behaviour in the dying one has its origin in continuous discomfort, mental, physical and spiritual. At times, too, the side effects of many medications including the painkillers, notably morphine, can alter mood and attitude.

Mood swings, irritability, confusion, forgetfulness,

displays of aberrant behaviour, and inability to recognise loved ones can occur, particularly in the case of brain tumours. Dementia may arise with advanced Aids in some cases. People with motor neurone syndrome may have fairly clear minds but just cannot speak. This is very difficult for us to accept and deal with as loved ones of the dying person. We must remember that the emotional and mental processes that the dying go through, dealing with deep feelings, and having to mourn their loss of family and loved ones as death approaches, have a huge effect on their mood. Realising this makes the mood swings more understandable.

Compassion is the paddle of the boat that takes us across the river of such days. The dying ones are proceeding on a journey which holds many new perceptions in their eyes.

No matter the religious belief, it is a journey into the unknown, into a space that nobody can control. People are generally very reluctant to face the unknown, so there can be a great deal of fear and anxiety at this stage, depending on the personality of the individual.

Overall: try not to take the negative attitudes of the dying personally. Instead, we should adjust our own attitudes in a spirit of love and understanding. This is a huge exercise in unconditional love for the family and carers. It is a tough lesson, all about giving with little possibility of return.

## The tricks of the dying

'He tries to manipulate me every chance he gets,' Nomvula confides. She touches on a common hazard for carers: being exposed to control and manipulation. This can hurt if not acknowledged and addressed. Dying does not mean that we don't still have a trick or two to play. At one level we have extra power because of our need for care and support. Gentle but firm response is required to set boundaries.

We have seen situations where the ill person has had entire squadrons of family members and friends running themselves ragged with ever-increasing demands and with unreasonable expectations. In one instance, Sandy derived a mischievous pleasure from setting those around her against one another. She would dispatch three people to run the same errand, driving everyone around her crazy until they caught her out. This happened partly because Sandy was bored and did not tell anyone how she felt. There were also unresolved issues, and this was her way of getting her own back before she died.

Outbursts of temper and moody sulking based on anger and resentment – often from unresolved agendas in relationships – can make life in already traumatic circumstances distressing and impossible. Patterns of behaviour, both good and bad, can be exacerbated in the face of serious illness and impending death.

Why not consider assistance from Hospice counsellors if

you have them in your area? Many others near you may also be trained in grief and bereavement counselling, such as social workers, psychologists, traditional healers, your priest or rabbi or imam, and counsellors from LifeLine. Their help is always available; it is just a matter of asking for it. There is no reason for anyone to stay a victim of verbal, mental or manipulative abuse from someone who is dying.

A caution here: Because of the abnormal circumstances, a pattern of over-control can arise and manifest itself without fanfare. Often it is only in hindsight that it dawns on us that abuse has happened. As reasonable human beings it is normal for us to want to bend over backwards to accommodate the notions and needs of the dying. Beware that the situation does not spin out of control and become backbreaking.

Distinguish between quality care and nursing and sheer slavery to will and command. The ability to say no or to leave the scene temporarily is vital for sanity's sake. The aim of the carer (often the partner) is to attend to the dying person, but not to do so in a way that encourages dependency. This is hard. You don't want to land up depriving the ill person of their own resources. The autonomy of all concerned is important. In this situation, the ill person can cleverly play one person off against another. Teamwork among family and friends, with the help of the appropriate counsellor and doctors, will give you the answer.

If the patient is signed up with a Hospice and an inpatient unit is available, the patient (and you) can enjoy a 14-day period of rest and respite. You could also consider outside nursing assistance to help take the pressure off the family.

The dying can be compliant and cooperative when faced with professional nurses, who are not emotionally involved. Yet they can also become petulant and resistant in a strange new environment. Turn to Hospice for guidance and help. Their services can make a real difference. Sometimes placement in a chronic illness institution may also be necessary. This needs careful discussion and planning with all concerned, including the ill person.

When we say that quality of life is vital, this includes not only the dying person but also all those around them. Voracious diseases such as cancer kill people, but should not be allowed to destroy healthy happy relationships. HIV/Aids is another burden that undermines and threatens the equilibrium in families, posing questions, anxieties and prejudices that cause a great deal of stress and fear. So, for quality of life in the family, keep things as light as possible. Above all, try not to take yourself too seriously. We touch on this again in Chapter 7, which discusses how carers can care for themselves.

# 5
# Accepting death

Illness attends me with relentless care.
My intimate maid, she heeds her task
to undress my soul, remove from me
*the outer clothing of my inner self.*

*Viv Stacey*

In the middle of the last century Elisabeth Kübler-Ross pioneered new attitudes and responses to the dying in Europe and America, as Dame Cecily Saunders did in the United Kingdom. Instead of being left behind screens and avoided on ward rounds, the terminally ill patient was spoken to and the range of other concerns the patient had was addressed.

The initial responses of denial, anger, bargaining, depression and acceptance that Kübler-Ross identified can be expected in the dying person. These stages clearly express the roller-coaster range of human feeling that the ill person and the family experience. Therapists have since reworked the idea, focusing on the impact of loss and the emotional withdrawal it causes. We agree with this description of mourning as consisting of four tasks:

- Accepting the reality of the loss
- Working through the pain of grief
- Adjusting to an environment in which the deceased is missing
- Emotionally relocating the deceased and moving on with life.[1]

### Accepting the reality of death

Whether we die in a natural disaster, an accident, violently at the hand of another, or quietly in bed – we are losing our life in the world. If we are conscious as we fail and die, we know we are losing all the links and bonds that give our life texture, colour, dimensions, value, meaning; and – as some people believe – we could be losing our very selves, coming to an end. This is a profound shock, a complete disruption of the way things are, probably nowhere near the things we normally prepare ourselves for.

Our response may well be to mourn for ourselves. There could be a distinct feeling of being cheated or stolen from, leading to anger, confusion and a sense of being very let down. The stronger our attachments, the more difficult it is to face losing them.

Anger and denial are the emotional states that hold

out the longest in the dying and the family. To talk about dying is somehow seen as bringing it on or selling out on hope. In some cultures there is a taboo against speaking in this way. That our mortality is an unchangeable part of our human existence is not something we like to be reminded of.

But underneath the camouflage of denial and resistance[2] is the reality of death and loss for both the patient and the surviving carer. We have to see the reality and accept it.

Anger is sometimes more easily expressed than the disappointment, sadness, and fear of the unknown that may underpin it. It can also contain the passion for life, the protest against suffering, and the despair at the loss of a future that flood into the consciousness of the person coping with a limited life span. The carefully thought-out plans for the future all get upturned and there is a sense of nothingness that seems to stretch out ahead like an endless desert. It is not uncommon for some ill people, fearing the burden they are to their family, frustrated with the changed life, and dealing with physical and spiritual pain, to consider suicide.

The dying person may choose to stay in a state of anger, which can poison the mind. It is important that others listen to outbursts and acknowledge the anger. Carers might be tempted to deflect the issue for their own peace of mind when they are already struggling and doing the best they can. But the anger belongs to the person who experiences it, and can hide other feelings more difficult to admit to or to express.

Displaced anger, if directed at the carers, can end up isolating the person further. Carers have the difficult, loving task of weathering the storm and staying as true companions, no matter what. In fact, explicit swearing or punching movements can be an outlet for the build-up of tension that anger causes – this dynamic should be understood and even welcomed at times.

A friend, James, asked to be taken in his wheelchair to the sea. He was carried to the water's edge where, with all the strength he could muster, he vented his feelings verbally as loud as he could to the waves. The wind was blowing, and the surf kept crashing relentlessly onto the beach. When all the emotion was spent, he was able to weep tears of healing. James left the beach that stormy afternoon purged and at peace, to die quietly a few days later. This was a great lesson to us, and a tactic we then used most effectively to help assuage our own grief at his loss.

Using massage or guided meditation can help release the energy that anger builds up in the muscles (see Chapters 8 and 9 below). Directing the anger to God in an exclamatory prayer is also useful. Allowing the anger to thaw into tears of exhaustion and frustration can bring a shift in the underlying emotions as well, so that people lose their fear and sorrow. The more complex and multi-layered the levels of fear are in the dying person, the more time will need to be spent in counselling.

## Pushing to understand

When faced with our mortality, whatever inner resources we have will be called upon. Our spirituality at this point will be the whole scope of experience within us, of how we have related to life and people over the years of our living. What have our social contracts, choices and attitudes made of us? In our dying, that inner reality is exposed to ourselves and others.

The questions that patients ask indicate the challenges that dying brings and how people honour life. Has my life had meaning? What have I accomplished? What unfinished business is there in my life? What forgiveness have I asked for or given? What do I need to confess? What haunts me from the past? What are the feelings I currently experience – regret, shame, guilt, sadness, emptiness, self-rejection, horror of the unknown, a sense of the absence of God, despair, betrayal? What does it mean for me to let go of my life but to trust the continuing influence of my life's purpose and destiny? What are the experiences and moments for which I am deeply grateful? What can bring me joy and contentment *now*? How can I show appreciation and love to those around me? Can I still respond to the gift of being alive?

A retired Anglican chaplain, Kay Espley,[3] taught in her training lectures that each patient's worldview is a mixture of religious background, education and personal experience. Where a person's religious beliefs are strong, the overriding desire is to search for meaning and purpose in suffering and see them as part of God's plan.

As we approach our death, it is likely that many of us will believe one of two things. We could believe that we quite literally return to the earth and that our death is the ending of a process of life that has no sequel. Otherwise, in terms of the major religions of the world, we could believe that we do have a continuing existence, in spiritual consciousness in a realm hidden from our sight and understanding. There are many variations and descriptions of this existence. They include the images of angels, paradise or heaven, and the idea of reconnecting with the ancestors or family who have died ahead of us.

As carers, taking the patient seriously involves suspending our own views of suffering and death. The dying need to find their own voice in response to these realities and others too. For some, love is mostly about sex, religion is an empty fantasy, and the only way to find meaning is through beauty, justice or humanitarian values. We might not agree, but we should uphold the dying and be open to what they are thinking. More than that, we need to adopt an attitude that releases the person who is dying from fear and anxiety around their experience of their mortality.

In spite of trauma, fear and grief, there are simple ways to transform the quality of life for all concerned into something extraordinary. The spiritual needs of the dying are basically to be loved, to be understood, to be respected, to be valued, to have some construct of meaning and hope. Certainly the first four we can supply without debate.

The life crisis of a terminal illness demands things from everyone that are beyond our ordinary resources. The struggle is to make sense of past experience and to relate to the new experience in a meaningful way. Our world changes and so we have lost some of what gave us our bearings before; but in the new situation there will be other factors – unexpected ones, surprises – waiting to provide meaning and purpose.

## Thinking of ending it all

Yet situations can and do arise where, in the mind of the one who is dying, suicide looks like a better option than sticking it out. Some patients, faced with increasing helplessness, physical disability and extreme pain, are drawn to the idea of bringing it all to a premature end. Their trend of thought needs to be seriously acknowledged and responded to. This is an uncomfortable ethical area, with a huge range of opinion quite beyond the scope of this book. In some places in the world, legal guidelines are in place for physician-assisted suicide (euthanasia). This debate still has to come before the South African parliament. While having a liberal Constitution, the strong underlying religious values in South Africa may well put brakes on any such legislation.

Peter describes a counselling session with a seriously ill patient who wanted to end his life. He had lived with his disease for five years. Peter said to him, 'Jack, by ending your life you give death more power than it already has over you.' His reply: 'By not ending my life I give this disease more power than it has already exercised over me. I want to see it defeated.' Peter found himself silenced. Jack could only hang on to the last shreds of his human dignity with great effort. He had wrestled with his conscience. With his resilient spirit, in the face of ravaging illness, he profoundly wanted to live or die on his own terms. When, shortly afterwards, he contracted pneumonia, he chose not to have antibiotics and died a few days later. His acquiescence in death was not entirely on death's terms alone.

A choice we do have available to us is to draw up a statement called a Living Will. A Living Will is an important document that asks the family and the medical team to stop treatments that prolong the life of the person who is in the process of dying, and to that extent gives them the moral right to do so. This document should be kept separately from your Last Will and Testament, and a copy given to the doctor in charge as well as to the primary carer, while you are still of sound mind.

A Living Will is a 'prickle-patch'. It does not authorise anybody to end your life, but is a moral request to end life-supporting treatments that prolong life and consequent suffering when you can no longer declare your wishes. Some primary next of kin can object strongly in this matter. Again, as we have upheld throughout our writings, it is wise and compassionate to respect the preference of the one suffering over and above the treasured opinions of others.

The Living Will Society provides a basic document that people can sign. This is an advanced instruction devised to stand as a declaration of non-consent to artificial life-support in the event of a person being unable to communicate when dying. It is wise to have three or more original copies signed when of sound mind and after careful consideration, in the presence of two witnesses. It is imperative to share this weighty decision with anyone who may have to implement it – this could be your attending doctor, primary carer, family or friends.

Contact details for the Living Will Society are included in the Contacts section at the end of this book. Their excellent website is easy to follow, with comprehensive information and sound advice. The mission statement of the society (also called 'Saves') declares that the Living Will

- saves suffering and pain
- saves anxiety for loved ones

- saves valueless prolongation of terminal illness
- saves existence without quality of life, and
- saves spending life savings unnecessarily.

**The dying child**

A child dying in the womb, at birth, or shortly afterwards, or in infancy, toddler stage or adolescence is a traumatic event for family members, requiring careful attention in grief management. For the children themselves, the fears and anxieties can be intense and the presence and reassurance of carers become crucial. The principles of non-abandonment and honesty are important when attending to a dying child.

The separating process is painful for the child, the parent and the siblings in different ways. Children dying can be encouraged to make memory boxes for the parent – collecting items, objects, letters, drawings that become gifts to the parent, gifts that are invested with the unique spirit of the child. This is also a way of saying, 'I existed'; 'I had my place in this family'; 'I will not be forgotten.'

Hospice in Cape Town has the resource 'About Me', which is a game a child plays with the parent or counsellor that helps them track the fears, needs and emotions that are difficult for them in the dying process. It expresses what they are experiencing without imposing the parents' fearful projections. Another resource available from Hospice is the book *Water Bugs and Dragonflies* by Doris

Stickney, and the 'Letter to a Child with Cancer'[4] by Elisabeth Kübler-Ross, written to a 9-year-old boy who had asked, 'What is life?', 'What is death?' and 'Why do young children have to die?' In simple language the letter relates the child to images in nature and gives an understanding of a Creator God who is present with us in the 'gamble of life' and who is in charge. She talks in this resource about being imprisoned in a cocoon and how our soul escapes into the form of the butterfly.

## Some positive attitudes to dying

Patch Adams – the doctor famous for the use of humour and clowning in the treatment of patients facing life-threatening illnesses – says that our attitude to our illness is our choice. If fear and anxiety rule us, then we will only see medical pathology and progression of disease. He challenges all of us – the medical profession, psychiatrists, patients and their families – to adopt a more holistic idea of mental health so that we can laugh and feel joy in the midst of trials. We can then see our troubles in a wider perspective and take them a bit more lightly. The humour helps to restore our inner balance and opens up other interpretations.[5]

A similar idea underlies the surgeon Bernie Siegal's books.[6] He appeals to the 'inner healer' in patients to come up with ideas about treatment so that the patients have a hand in shaping the procedures they must endure.

By engaging people's wisdom and humour, he guides them to a fuller appreciation of what it means to be human.

The popular book *Tuesdays with Morrie* by Mitch Albom[7] also protests against the dehumanising process of illness and praises the staying power of the human spirit. This book records the power implicit in a life that is ending and its capacity to rekindle hope and love in the face

Anneline Malebo, the former lead singer of the group Joy, bestrode the stages of the world until she was infected by the HIV virus as a result of rape.[8] Seriously ill with full-blown Aids, she was mostly bedridden – but until her death in 2002 her dignity and courage still shone through. Anneline believed that, as long as she sang, her disease would be unable to kill her spirit. She sang her famous song 'Paradise Road' at the opening of the St Luke's Hospice ward at Conradie Hospital, Cape Town, in May 2002. Her voice rang out strong and clear:

Come with me to Paradise Road
This way please I'll carry your load
This you won't believe

Come with me to Paradise Skies
Look outside and open your eyes
This you must believe

of inevitable death. What survives people's death is a fragrance of their personality, a memory of them, and an experience of sharing their life and dying that brings forth new life. Given that emphasis, dying does not have to be traumatic and depressing.

To be confronted with a terminal diagnosis requires that we settle our own understanding and attitude to our mortality. The major religions speak of a passageway through death to paradise or heaven or some alternative experience hidden from our sight and understanding. In those terms, death is seen as a point of transformation or transition from one level of existence to another.

One assumption is that on earth we vibrate at a lower frequency, as it were, from those in the non-physical world. When we step outside our body we are in an altogether different dimension, and our frequency changes. The Dalai Lama describes death as 'life, changing clothes'. He also says, 'Life and death are the changes. In the clear light and after death these movements fall below the clear light state.'[9]

Others echo this belief. Thich Nhat Hahn says, 'In Zen we like to ask the question "What did your face look like before your grandmother was born?" Ask yourself this question and you will begin to see your own continuation. You will see that you have always been there. The moment of your conception is a moment of continuation, of manifesting in another form. If you keep looking, you'll see that instead of birth and death, there is the continuing transformation.'[10]

The greatest challenge to our mental grasp of death is the question of what happens to our consciousness, which holds the secrets of our personality and life essence. The questions people ponder over are whether that consciousness and the memories associated with it in the brain disappear with the disintegration of the brain at the time of death.

David Lorrimer, formerly director of the Scientific and Medical Network, argues that the brain produces consciousness and therefore is understood at death to be either extinguished or *filtering* that consciousness into a wider state. There are changes and expansions at the moment of death into that other dimension. His quantified research challenges the idea that memories stored in the brain disintegrate with the death of the brain. He cites verified evidence of children who remember events that happened to others. This suggests that human existence is far more profoundly mysterious and spiritual than is commonly assumed in the West.[11]

The psychologist and author Robert Johnson argues that suffering can be a catalyst for true transformation of attitudes and lifestyle, if processed honestly and courageously.

Seen in that spirit, dying could be the supreme stage for inner growth on earth.

Dying can teach us how to live. Beverley Rycroft confronted her mortality in the context of chemo-therapy treatments. Here is her statement:

I was living a life excessive in every sense other than spiritual. Excessively busy, excessively preoccupied with what others might think, how I could earn more money, possessions, clothes I wanted to wear, things to own. My desires for material possessions and the admiration of others were paramount. My spiritual life was a cracked, dry riverbed.

The diagnosis of a life-threatening disease and the dire treatment proposed shattered that dishonest life. That first night – the night of my diagnosis – I lay awake in the darkness looking straight into the face of the eternal mystery of death. I wanted only one thing – to be granted the privilege of living to see my grandchildren one day. Nothing else mattered. I could have walked out of my beautiful house, left my car, my books, my TV, my new computer – all the things I had put so much energy into acquiring and maintaining. I saw finally that all those things were finite and destructible. In the end they would wear away, break down, fall apart and disintegrate.

Even my children and my husband – and this was the hardest part – would one day be faced with death. I realised that even my family, the most precious, most fiercely loved of all, would have to be released from my grasp before I could begin to heal. The only thing that could not be destroyed, could not be X-rayed or removed or injected or operated on or cremated was my soul. Strapped into yet another tunnel-shaped machine for X-ray examination of my internal organs, I distracted myself by wondering whether the day would ever come when people would examine their soul in the same way. 'Well, Mrs Jones, I'm afraid we've found signs of degenerative greed and avarice in your inner soul. Unfortunately there is also envy and hatred that's spread to your heart. We are going to give it the best treatment we can and see what happens.'

The potter, they say, can smash the clay. The clay out of which God formed me was flung to the ground and shattered. Yet with painstaking slowness, God set about helping me pick up those fragments, those needle-sharp shards, and fit them all back together again. With infinite and extra-ordinary love God helped me rebuild my soul. He gave back to me a supreme gift – the only thing medical science will not touch. Like Hans Christian Andersen's little tin soldier, I was led through desolation and danger and flung finally into a fire from which my soul alone emerged intact.

# Notes

1 J William Worden, *Grief Counselling and Grief Therapy: A Handbook for the Mental Health Practitioner*. London: Routledge, 1991. 10.

2 We are indebted for this phrase to Ganga Stone, who in turn drew the idea of seeing through camouflage to reality from a remarkable story. A man was employed by the army to fly low over the countryside spotting tanks and small aircraft that were concealed under camouflaged cloth below. 'You see,' he said, 'I am colour-blind, so I can't see the camouflage – I can only see the shape of the thing as it is.' *Start the Conversation: The Book about Death You Were Hoping to Find*. New York: Warner, 1996. 4.

3 Formerly Anglican chaplain at Groote Schuur Hospital in Cape Town, and a course educator in clinical pastoral training.

4 The letter comes at the end of her book *The Tunnel and the Light*.

5 This brief outline is based on his widely known views, and his comments to us in Cape Town in 2002.

6 We refer particularly to *Living, Loving and Healing*. London: Aquarian/Thorsons, 1993; and *Love, Medicine and Miracles*. London: Arrow, 1986.

7 *Tuesdays with Morrie: An Old Man, A Young Man, and Life's Greatest Lesson*. London: Warner, 1997.

8 Story adapted from *St Luke's Hospice News*, August 2002.

9 Quoted by Rob Nairn in a lecture given at the Buddhist Centre, Kenilworth, Cape Town, in November 1994 as part of a symposium on Dying.

10 *No Death, No Fear: Comforting Wisdom for Life*. Riverhead, 2003.

11 *Thinking Beyond the Brain*. Floris, 2001. 7.

# 6
# Mourning

*Squeezing Life's Summer*

You feel the days closing
slipping from your grasp
like that last hour on the dance floor
before the morning light.
The last game of the year
one more innings to go
the final walk-in with the bowler
bringing the season to a close.
Saying farewell to an old matc
one you knew so well
thinking of the fun times
the warmth in you still tells.
Stroking the brow of an ebbing friend
The sadness of a fading farewell
you cannot think of a life without –
yet you know there will.

*Tim Wood*

## Saying goodbye to a life
We have said that the dying are likely to mourn for themselves, feel cheated and stolen from, and so grow angry and

confused. The stronger their attachments, the more difficult it is for people to face losing them. This is equally true for those being left behind. When someone deeply loved dies, or even where there were conflicted relationships with the person, the emotional aftermath can be overwhelming.

It is vital to acknowledge these feelings: only then can we readjust to life and other relationships. The loss is keenly felt because we have to disinvest our emotional connection to a large extent – the companionship will just become one in the memory, or an imaginary one that we might maintain for a long time afterwards. We may have to abandon the way we lived before, and certain hopes and plans too. These ruptures are hard to endure, and leave the grieving person feeling isolated even in company. Nobody, it seems, is able to understand the void that is left inside, the emptiness outside, and the inconsolable heart.

The pain of grief is felt in the psyche. If ignored, this can affect the body, causing physical illness. This was recognised in seventeenth-century England, where one of the listed causes of death was 'Griefe'. We still talk of dying of a broken heart, acknowledging the physical strain. Attending to the pain means having to acknowledge the suffering, talk to a counsellor perhaps, and come to terms with a changed life. No wonder so many people prefer to bottle up their feelings, sometimes for years – but they do so at great cost emotionally and physically.

## The Valley of Shadows

As we link our hands
You bring my chattering mind
My cluttered thoughts
From churning water to stillness.

The bed holds you lightly.
Your body caught between
Fighting and forsaking
Unties the rope
That holds the boat of your soul
To this shore.

We gaze in silence
As the river widens
I try to find the echoes, the words
That bridge the chasm
Between us
Around us
Within us.

The nurse checks the syringe-driver
And moistens your cracked lips.
Does medication ease the way for your soul's crossing?

Pulsing in me – your unanswered questions.
Your scattered memories
Of love and betrayal.
Of ecstasy and tears.

Your fears and purposes
Shift into a current
No oar can hold.

What is this steep bank?
This edge? This precipice?
This threshold of no return?
This turbulent water?
The river of the shadow?

The passage slackens
The lines between your head,
heart and breath.
The boat takes in water.
The river drowns your vitality
And quietly mocks faith's firm finalities
That the crossing is sure.

Songs not of this earth
Filter mystery across the water
Through no-thingness
Lifting the engulfing mists.

The bedside clock
Flickerprints
The eddy of time
Measured on my side of the bank.

Your hand hold loosens
To a fingertip touch.

*Peter Fox*

So the challenge, once the tears have dried, is to move on, rethinking priorities and reshaping life. Principles and what people value come to the fore. One of the realities of working through adversity is that we can arrive at an understanding of true spirituality – how to live our life. (Religions are natural outgrowths of this, which some of us live by and others don't. Your quest for inner truth may well be in other terms.) The material for this exploration is often the unconscious elements in our minds and hearts; what is hidden will find a way of coming to the surface and needing to be dealt with. This could be a time when you discover the strength and resilience of your spirit.

We can differentiate between spirituality and religion. While religion draws from spirituality, for most of us it remains only a part of our spirituality. A commentator has this to say:

'Spirituality' relates to our souls. It involves that deep inner essence of who we are. It is an openness to the possibility that the soul within each of us is somehow related to the Soul of all that is. Spirituality is what happens to us that is so memorable we cannot forget it, and yet we find it difficult to talk about because words fail to describe it.

Spirituality is the act of looking for meaning in the very deepest sense, and looking for it in the way that is most authentically ours. Now 'religion', on the other hand, works in a different way. While spirituality is necessarily very personal, religion is more communal . . . Religion has to do with collecting and consolidating and unifying.

Spirituality is a far broader concept, for it refers to all the ways we invest life with meaning, including theistic beliefs, philosophies and ideologies. Spirituality is universal: while individuals may or may not have religious beliefs (i.e. adhere to an organised set of doctrines), spirituality is inherent.

Spirituality is about the way the life of desire in us moves to accomplish things. We create, we give compassion, we contribute knowledge and wisdom. It is the song that is uniquely our own . . . Dying does not change all these realities. Dying can become the deepest spiritual experience of a lifetime.[1]

The terrible sorrow and lonely hollowness must be acknowledged. There is no pill or external treatment that can ease the emptiness and pain. In time and with creative attention, such a state can fruitfully lead to us reviewing our lives. Loneliness can be transformed into inner stillness, a tranquil solitude away from the clamour of our scheduled lives, a place of rest.

New activities have to be broached deliberately. After a while, people in mourning could consider pursuing a new hobby, another work skill, fresh social contact and commitments. For some, a new relationship with nature begins – going on mountain, beach or country walks, joining a botanical society, learning about plants or animals, gardening, which they might not have done before. These are ways to reconnect with life in a purposeful fashion. They help to restore a sense of equilibrium.

For people in grief or any other stress, domestic pets can be a great source of comfort.

If you are bereaved and haven't a pet already, this might be the time to get one. Animals can be good quiet company and they have intuition. In various ways that are not at all imaginary, they really can make you feel better – for example, a cat purrs at the same frequency as ultrasound therapy, which helps to set broken bones.

## Support for children

Children experience sorrow and loss intensely. They are forced to cope with changes and threats to their emotional and physical stability, and to their daily routine. They need to be encouraged to speak about what is held deeply within them. This can only be done in a climate of trust and safety. It is vital to take children seriously and not to overlook or ignore them in their suffering.

Teachers and parents need to be sensitive so as not to single out the individual in a way that draws undue attention to them, causing embarrassment and loss of face with their peers. On the other hand, to ignore the distress in a child and discourage giving any attention is equally unhelpful.

Sometimes parents can't cope with the children's feelings because they are hardly coping with their own. Some families have a culture of silence and closing rank, insisting that these coping mechanisms are sufficient within the family circle. But children need to be included, and must not meet with silence. The process of watching a close relative die could be the most difficult thing a child has ever been through. They are handicapped by their youth and lack of life experience. Communicate with them in a gentle but honest way. This will assure them that support and answers to their questions are constantly available. Shielding children from grief when they need to be included in the mourning process may, as time passes, prove more harmful than helpful.

Funerals or memorial services are a time when families can mourn and comfort one another openly, and also honour and celebrate the life of the deceased loved one. No child should be forced to attend the ceremony, but if children are old enough to understand what is happening they could benefit greatly. Give children the choice, let them decide if they want to attend. This gives them an active role in the family events.

If children wish to attend or participate in some way, they need to be heard and supported. They may choose to read a poem or a story, light a candle, play a musical instrument or request a special piece of music – perhaps a song or a hymn – to be sung. At one funeral I remember the grandchildren drawing with crayons on the wooden coffin of their grandfather during the funeral service.

If you are very upset yourself, it can be wonderfully healing to cry with any child in your care. A good weep is cathartic when so much pain is bottled up in us. It is the release that soothes us when there is no other balm available. Crying with the child brings balance and normality to the situation. It also shows the child that it is quite okay to cry even when you are a grown-up.

Children whose loved ones have died are bereaved like anyone else. They must not be deprived inadvertently of the opportunity to mourn their loss. Unwanted grief can cause havoc in relationships in later years, and also in attitudes to the self and the world.

Consider involving an appropriate relative, social worker or other counsellor if a child seems to be battling with grief. There are games children can play that help them access their feelings of loss. Writing, and drawing in art therapy, are other very successful ways to bring out repressed feelings. Age-sensitive counselling will include understanding the child or adolescent's needs at that stage of their lives. Some children and teenagers are more resilient than others; it depends on their upbringing and personalities.

Sometimes children are spoken to harshly, almost cruelly, in times of grief because of the defence mechanisms that mourning adults adopt to protect their own feelings. Our hope is that, whether you are a professional, lay carer or relative, you will find yourself able to speak to the children gently, wisely and with love. They are young impressionable souls, and they need all the care you can give them.

One of the most frequently encountered feelings expressed by the bereaved is a sense that time just passed too quickly while that person was alive. It is so important to make the most of the time we have – and that means living in the present. As the poet William Blake says:

To see a world in a grain of sand
And heaven in a wild flower.
Hold infinity in the palm of your hand
And eternity in an hour.

## Note

1   J Miller, 'Spirituality'. Paper presented to the conference on Transformational Grief, in Burnsville, USA, November 1994.

# 7
# Care for the carers

Sometimes when I cry
I feel as though it has
                just rained,
             leaving me fresh,
             able to continue
             once again . . .

*Donni and George Betts*

## Hospice help
It is hard to separate the needs of the dying person from those of the family and carers.

Carers have needs of their own that are very different from the patient's, and so quality care of the patient does not always cater for those at the bedside. Patient-focused care should also nurture those who are involved in it.

There are times when things just get too much. Some carers feel awkward about admitting to those close to them that they feel overwhelmed. But you don't have to struggle on alone as an individual carer or a group. The community around you has other resources, and if you have a Hospice in your area this is probably your first port of call. Hospice focuses as much on the needs of the immediate family as on those of the dying. In your daily efforts, you need not be alone.

Part of the function of Hospice is that it provides relief to the exhausted carers, who carry the physical and emotional responsibility of caring for a dying person. Often the patient is already aware of how demanding their care is, and the load of responsibility on their caregivers. Nobody then has to explain why relief arrangements are being made.

Patients can be admitted for symptom control, family relief, or terminal care. It is helpful if the hospital or doctor makes early referrals to Hospice. This allows the ill person and the family to experience the benefit of the nursing and counselling. Hospice is also valuable in providing a place where the feelings of the ill person about being a burden can be heard and discussed.

Hospice care offers wide support, usually with a team comprising a doctor, professional nurses, physiotherapists, occupational therapists, social workers, spiritual counsellors, and volunteers. The support structure enables the family as well as the patient to embrace the approaching death as the end of a journey that has quality and dignity, in an atmosphere of compassion. Everyone – in body, mind and spirit – can then accompany the dying person in final partnership. This makes it possible to speak of 'a good death'.

When the patient is admitted to Hospice, the caregiving family members are able to replenish lost energy. Don't underestimate the all-absorbing nature of caring for a dying person. It challenges everyone's imagination and creative resources.

## Other outside support

In some instances the carer needs to continue working and earning a living. Finding a support group of other carers in similar situations could offer emotional containment for the stresses that caregiving involves.

If there is a need to talk anonymously to skilled counsellors, LifeLine provides telephonic and face-to-face service. Their confidential, skilled help is given free of charge.

You may sometimes need to share the situation with someone outside the family as pressure builds up. Feelings of guilt often paralyse the carer into not expressing frustration, despair and anger. Here a trusted friend or colleague can help.

## Nurturing your body

When you experience stiffness and pain, particularly in the neck, shoulder and back, your body is asking you for a good massage. This is a wonderful way to manage stress and tension directly. Explore the avenues of chiropractic, body stress release and acupuncture outlined below, or aromatherapy, reflexology, therapeutic body massage, reiki and physiotherapy described briefly in Chapter 8. All these treatments are effective, so take your pick.

Eating simply but adequately helps maintain energy and resilience. Prepare your favourite food. Acknowledge, then put aside, any feelings of guilt that you are enjoying this food while the one you are nursing is unable to do so. Fresh air, exercise and enough sleep are priorities.

Nursing your patient may injure you physically as you lift the person, carry heavy weights, and have to use your body in awkward ways. There are several avenues to explore for maintaining your health, releasing tension, and helping to clear up any physical damage:

- **Chiropractic** is a health care discipline utilising adjustments and other manual techniques aimed at restoring joint function and assisting the body's healing function.
- **Body stress release**, gentle in its application, is similar to chiropractic. This technique is designed to aid the body to release its stored-up tension by activating reflex points to the joints and muscles and thereby restoring balance and ease.
- **Acupuncture** is a Chinese discipline that uses needles along the meridians of the body. This practice is designed to unblock *chi* (or energy, as it is

known in the West) along all the meridians, to promote harmony and balance in the body, mind and spirit – and thus good health.

## Taking time out, and other self-care

If frustrations and anger start building up, it is time to take a break from each other. Even while you're on the spot, count to ten and breathe deeply before lashing back in defence or retaliation, or in projecting your own pain about the impending loss. Try to observe and understand the source of the reactions you meet. This can be an opportunity to gain new insight.

Count your blessings. You do have some, you know! And look on the light side whenever you can. Here is a litany for carers, written by one who knows:

For the day that starts and ends well,
*We are thankful.*
For the medications that work – most of the time,
*We are thankful.*
For the hand that is steady and the foot that
    can step,
*We are thankful.*
For the struggle that ends in success,
*We are thankful.*
For the smile that cracks that mask,
*We are thankful.*

For the nights of healing rest,
*We are thankful.*
For shared communication,
*We are thankful.*
For those who understand,
*We are thankful.*
For memories of days past, and hope for tomorrow,
For love that sustains us both,
*We are, most of all, thankful.*[1]

Exhaustion affects every side of life – mental, emotional and physical. Making time to relax in nature, go to theatres or movies, or just hang out with friends helps to give you back your balance. A long relaxing soak in a hot bath, an invigorating shower, a good cry, a brisk walk, a visit to the hairdresser, are other ways to restore yourself. These are welcome breaks that you need for sanity's sake.

As far as possible, avoid draining and negative situations and people. It may help if you give up reading the newspapers and viewing television newscasts and programmes that are distressing. Try to focus instead on the beauty around you and good things within the range of your loved one's experience. Shifting to the positive is crucial as the family prioritises the important over the less important. It is a form of inner stocktaking that can deepen the soul's response to love and life.

Nature, sunsets and beautiful music are great soothers for frayed nerves and heartache.

The Chinese poet Li Po writes:

If you were to ask me why I dwell among green
    mountains
I should laugh silently; my soul serene.
The peach blossom follows the moving water;
There is another heaven and earth beyond the
    world of men.[2]

**Nine tips for carers**
The Hospice of Lancaster County, Pennsylvania, offers this advice to family carers:

- Choose to take charge of your life. Don't let your loved one's illness or disability always take the centre stage.
- Be good to yourself. You are doing a very hard job and you deserve some quality time just for you.
- When people offer help, accept the offer and suggest specific things they can do.
- Educate yourself about your loved one's condition. Information is empowering.
- There is a difference between caring and doing. Be open to technologies and ideas that promote your loved one's independence.

- Trust your instincts; most of the time they will lead you in the right direction.
- Grieve for your losses: but allow yourself to dream new dreams.
- Stand up for your rights as a caregiver and citizen.
- Seek support from other caregivers. There is great strength in knowing that you are not alone.[3]

## Notes

1   'A Caregiver's Litany' by Camilla Hewson Flintermann, from handout material prepared by the Hospice of Lancaster County, Lancaster, PA, available at St Luke's Hospice in Cape Town.

2   Translated by Sam Hamill. *The Enlightened Heart: An Anthology of Sacred Poetry*, ed Stephen Mitchell. 31.

3   Taken from handout material prepared by the Hospice of Lancaster County, PA.

# 8
# Supportive therapies for the dying

Darling, do you remember
The man you married? Touch me,
Remind me who I am.

*Stanley Kunitz*

## Guidance by the dying

To the dying person we say: Remember this is your own body and ultimately you are responsible for every single choice you make as to what you allow to be injected, rubbed or spooned into it. Open yourself and your family to all the other options for health and disease management. Never forget that you have the power of choice.

Gently but firmly refuse to be coerced into any decisions on the spur of an emotional moment. Question treatments that are highly aggressive, and be sure to find out exactly what the side effects will be. Discuss in depth with your physician what you are trying to achieve in a terminal state. Honest communication on all sides – the patient, the carers and the family – is imperative for good management.

Take part in considering new remedies. A time of dying can still be one of learning new skills. It is said that the Greek philosopher Socrates was in prison awaiting death when another prisoner read the works of a poet to him. Socrates expressed the desire to learn the poem off by heart. 'What for? You are soon going to die.' Socrates responded, 'At least I will die knowing one more thing.'

We say to the carers: Those who have lived through ill health and the discomforts of treatment for a long time tend to grow apathetic and resign themselves to whatever others prescribe. Sometimes people in that state think that when they comment on their condition they sound as if they are seeking attention or else are being trivial. Exhaustion plays its part too in their inability to communicate changes in pain and other symptoms.

But the dying should not be stoics, suffering in silence. Share the options of therapy with them and help them to give their views. Communication is possible in any caring situation – with hands, words and eyes. Ask gentle questions and encourage them to express their pain and other bothersome symptoms. Never impose any form of alternative therapy without permission or request from the dying person.

## General points on therapy

Pain control is probably the most important need of all, and can be achieved by the appropriate use of analgesia along with other remedies. Many alternative therapies, if used responsibly, can provide comfort and add quality to daily life.

In the fields that we explore here, some families may not be able to afford professional treatment and so they would forfeit these gentle therapies. People then also feel humiliated and helpless when they don't use them. We suggest that you enlist the help of qualified practitioners for advice on treatment and a lesson or two in basic techniques. With that supervision, you can practise these skills yourself.

Do not impose any therapies on the one dying because they are 'good for you'. Avoid practitioners who are not respectful of this ethic, and also be wary of professionals who are prejudiced against methods of treatment other than their own.

A word of caution: There are the odd unscrupulous practitioners in every field, so be careful whom you choose. Check that the professionals you are considering are properly registered to practise their chosen discipline by referring first to the Allied Health Professionals Council of South Africa or the Health Professions Council of South Africa. The latter is an umbrella body over the new, separate Medical and Dental Councils; it sets and maintains the standards for health care in South Africa, and every health professional must be registered with it. The contact details are listed in the Contacts section at the end of this book

As a background to all therapy and care, try to create an atmosphere of calm and peace in the patient's room, so that it becomes a sanctuary rather than a sick bay. This will benefit everyone, and so will the tranquillity that the therapies can bring if properly applied.

Here follows a brief introduction to some therapies that could benefit those who are dying. It's a good idea to join a library – belonging to one is free – so that you can read relevant books on these subjects. We list some useful titles in the References section at the end of this book.

## Aromatherapy and massage

Taken together, this is the art of gentle massage with the aid of essential oils. These oils are readily available at most pharmacies and health stores. A word of caution: essential oils are strong. Belief that all these derivatives of plants are harmless is wrong and can be dangerous. If you are unsure how to use the oils and need further advice, consult a qualified aromatherapist.

Always allow the ill person to test an aroma before using essential oils, as some can provoke a negative reaction. Be cautious about the substance you use for massage. Most people who have had chemotherapy, radiation and other treatments have a damaged sense of smell and taste. Often the sense of smell has become ultra-sensitive to certain odours and this can induce severe bouts of nausea and vomiting, so don't just impose what you might think is a helpful aroma. Ask first.

Observe carefully as you massage. Working with physical touch, you will often be able to notice changes in symptoms and conditions quite clearly, even visibly. Fluctuation in mood and emotions may be extremely apparent. Keep on encouraging the dying to discuss their state and to draw attention to any problems. Report these changes clearly and accurately to the doctor and the other members of the caring team so that they can respond.

Gentle massaging of hands and feet is generally welcome – touch is a vital part of a good care routine. If appropriate, use one or two drops of lavender, neroli or mandarin in 10 ml of carrier oil. Sue says:

> In my 24 years of experience I have found these oils to be the least invasive for a body whose vital organs are rapidly failing. Most other oils I have found to be too strong for an already damaged liver and kidneys.
>
> The wellbeing of the patient is all-important, so I do not believe in adding any further ingredients to an overloaded dying body.
>
> Excellent use can be made of the essential

oils in burners. A drop or two on a handkerchief works well. In order to aid rest, a couple of drops of lavender on the pillow and bed sheet make a pleasant difference.

These are useful essential oils for the burner:
- Lavender has calming, soothing and balancing properties, and freshness.
- Neroli is helpful for shock and distress
- Mandarin is gentle and soothing for the digestive system.
- Grapefruit has uplifting qualities.
- Peppermint is effective for nausea and overriding cooking and other unpleasant odours, where the system has become oversensitive and is sometimes provoked into bouts of vomiting.
- Lemongrass is a strong fragrance. Apart from being pleasantly astringent, it overrides other nauseating odours.
- Eucalyptus has properties that fight bacteria, viruses and fungi. It works well in burners or as a room spray.

In the terminal stages of some cancers, aromatherapy is actually damaging and should be avoided. The skin often becomes paper-thin, exceptionally dry, flaky and sensitive. Body hair will have been compromised as well by the after-effects of chemotherapy and radiotherapy.

Also, the skin is affected as the body simply breaks down. Bleeding under the skin and easy bruising are common. Where there is lymphoedema of the arms, hands, legs and feet (depending on the part of the body affected) there is a painful build-up of liquid, resulting in very stretched sore skin. In some instances gentle massage can help, using olive oil, aqueous cream or a good lanolin-cream baby product. Massage in such cases is not normally recommended, however, and if it is done it should be supervised by a qualified therapist in conjunction with the health care professional.

Where massage is contra-indicated because of dramatic weight loss, adverse skin conditions and general areas of great discomfort, just hold the feet gently around the ankles, or the hands around the wrists, and sit quietly with the one in your care. You can also gently rest your hands on the nape of the neck, forehead and temples.

As death approaches, oils such as frankincense, cedarwood, bergamot and melissa aid the process of transition.[1] These are best used in a burner in the room. A drop or two of rose oil on a handkerchief is comforting.

## Reiki

Reiki is a Japanese word that means 'universal life energy'.[2] A Japanese doctor, Mikao Usui, conceived this method of healing in the mid-nineteenth century. It is a gentle and pleasant way to induce a sense of calm, balance and relaxation by releasing emotional blockages.

This simple method of holding the hands just above the body, moving them over the body without friction, allows the *ki* (life force or energy) to flow through the practitioner's hands to the recipient. This gentle art releases calm and relaxes and touches our whole being. It is well worth having a reiki practitioner in for a session or two to demonstrate how this can be done. Learning to do reiki does not require any special skill – everyone has the natural ability to use their hands in a healing way. (Healing in the context of the dying does not mean curing but alleviating the person's condition in some way, bringing relief.)

## Reflexology

Reflexology is the art of massaging the feet and hands, working on the reflex points that connect to all parts of the body. This technique restores balance, releases tension, and promotes a sense of wellbeing and relaxation. This may be helpful in the terminal phase of illness. It is, however, not wise to stimulate these points too much. Gentle stroking of the hands and feet is probably more appropriate. Discuss this with a trained reflexologist.

## Bach flower remedies

There are 38 essences, the best known and most widely used being Rescue Remedy. They do not take the place of skilled medical attention, nor were they designed to do so, but they are highly effective. For those unfamiliar with them, here is a little background on their origin and use.

Dr Edward Bach discovered this non-invasive method of treatment during the 1930s while practising as a renowned physician in Harley Street, London. He was also a qualified homeopath and bacteriologist. His mission was to find simple remedies so that lay people could treat themselves and their families simply and safely. He discovered these essences, all from plants, over a period of time and put them to many a test.

Their action is gentle, working on a person's mood. They do not interfere with other medications being taken simultaneously, and are non-toxic, and safe to administer to children. They are also non-addictive. Case histories and treatments are well documented. A good book to read is *The Illustrated Handbook of the Bach Flower Remedies* by Philip Chancellor, and you can also contact the Dr Edward Bach Centre in the UK. Details of both are given at the end of this book.

**Rescue Remedy:** Dr Bach developed this formula for use in emergencies and times of crisis that go on for long periods. The remedy contains five of his 38 essences: Star of Bethlehem for shock, Impatiens for tension and mental stress, Cherry Plum for desperation and fear of losing the mind, Clematis for bemused out-of-body states, and Rock Rose for terror and panic.

This remedy is widely available from health shops and pharmacies. It is prepared as tablets and as a liquid tincture – the latter seems more effective. The original remedies imported from the UK are in concentrated form; be warned that some health shops make up their own version from the originals, which is dodgy, to say the least. We refer here only to the remedies packed in the UK.

To use the tincture, fill a 50 ml dropper bottle with still spring water and add 12 drops of the concentrated remedy. Initially add three drops of this mixture to a glass of water to be sipped frequently until the person grows calmer. Then reduce the sipping to every 15 minutes increasing to half an hour, according to the person's condition. Used over longer periods, give three drops of the prepared remedy in a teaspoon of water four times a day. If the person is unconscious or unable to sip water, use Rescue Remedy undiluted to moisten the lips, temples, and pulse points on the wrists. Everyone involved with the dying person would do well on frequent doses of Rescue Remedy themselves.

**Walnut** is useful as the time of death approaches and can be added to the Rescue Remedy. A 'link breaker' used in times of dramatic change, it helps to calm the dying person as death approaches. Those in close touch may also benefit from it as the time of death draws near, and afterwards too as they adjust to the new life without their loved one.

**Olive** is the remedy for exhaustion, both mental and physical. It helps relieve that state of being exhausted to the point of weeping that can be caused by days or months of suffering, for the dying one; and for the carer, by the long periods of nursing the dying person under demanding conditions.

Option 1: To a jug of water add 10 drops of either or both love and walnut remedies (they can be administered together). Pour out a glassful, to be sipped at frequent intervals throughout the day.

Option 2: Fill a 25 ml bottle with filtered still water. Add two drops of the olive tincture. Take five drops of this mixture on the tongue or in a little water every two to four hours.

## Homeopathy

In the eighteenth century Samuel Hahnemann explored and formalised this special system of medicine as we know it today in the West. It is a gentle but highly effective way of medicating the sick by stimulating the body to heal itself, and so it also strengthens the immune system. Although it is a complete system in its own right, it can be used safely alongside conventional drugs. Here the advice of a good practitioner would be helpful. A homeopath can prescribe the most effective potencies so that dosages are not rendered useless by the action of other medicines being taken at the time.

The remedies work with the body's natural rhythms. This is an important point in their favour when treating the terminally ill patient. Some of the unpleasant symptoms arising from chemotherapy and radiotherapy can be alleviated homeopathically. The patient can experience a better quality of daily life and improved immunity against common viruses that would lead to further infection. Homeopathy treats the person in a holistic way, not simply addressing the obvious physical symptom only. When choosing a remedy, the attitude, frame of mind and emotional symptoms are part of the consideration. This form of treatment can be particularly helpful for states of fear, anxiety and depression, and for mood swings.

While there are many books available and many over-the-counter preparations, it is better to seek the help of an experienced homeopath. Everyone is unique, and there are many remedies for any one complaint – the aim being to choose the one that best suits both the person and the complaint. Then the beauty of this excellent system of medicine is likely to be felt as the patient experiences relief from symptoms together with a deeper sense of wellbeing.

If homeopathy is used, bear in mind that some aromatherapy oils can counteract the medicines because of their powerful fragrance and effect. Peppermint, camphor, eucalyptus and menthol are particularly strong. Chamomile can also interfere with certain remedies. Make informed choices, catering always for what is most needed.

Pain control is the most important process of all and can be achieved by the appropriate use of analgesia along with many other remedies.

## Physiotherapy

As well as being beneficial for the patient, this is another way to address the sore and stiff neck, back and body that the carer may suffer when looking after a bedridden person. It includes the technique of massage along with ultrasound and other aids that can bring relief. The physiotherapist's skills often improve physical movement and enhance lung function.

## Keeping up comfort and appearance

Along with these options, it is highly therapeutic to provide comfort and maintain self-worth and dignity. Hair and beards, toenails and fingernails are an intrinsic part of quality care routine.

Find a hairdresser who is equipped for home visits and prepared to come. Discuss attractive but practical styles and cuts that will suit the condition and circumstances best. Well-styled hair makes washing and drying easier in awkward surroundings.

Shaving can be made easier by using a battery-operated razor. Using a normal razor can be hazardous for the untrained hand, however willing the carer. Cuts and razor nicks add to discomfort and possible infection. Apply a gentle moisturiser to the face after cleaning or shaving, as the skin is almost always dry.

Heavy night-sweats and general perspiration, particularly in hot weather, make daily showering, bathing, bed-bathing and shampooing part of the essential routine.

Troublesome toenails, ingrown toenails and general foot discomfort need regular attention. A pedicure and manicure prevent long, sharp nails from scratching or catching on bedclothes, and feet from discomfort in shoes or slippers. As the body fails, nails can thicken and discolour or become paper-thin and fragile. Clear or cheerfully coloured nail varnish makes a difference.

Minimal but imaginative use of base and make-up works wonders for the self-image and esteem of the ill person. As far as possible and without causing excessive discomfort, help to keep the patient clean and presentable.

One of the greatest gifts to give a dying person is the opportunity to look well manicured, clean, and as attractive as possible. This simple act restores dignity when the body feels so ugly. The lack of control over normal body functions is already humiliating, so these small gestures are a great lifter of melancholy souls.

Attractive cotton pyjamas, shawls and scarves hide a multitude of disfigurements such as swellings and bloating. Scarves cleverly tied around a head made bald by treatment are most attractive, and are cooler and more comfortable than wigs.

A long towelling or cotton dressing gown and comfortable slippers are a help. Several changes of clean clothing and bed linen need to be on hand, as these items soil frequently as the body fails.

By attending to such details, in the midst of death we are still honouring the body.

> And when the day arrives for the last leaving
>   of all,
> And the ship that never returns to port is ready
>   to go,
> You will find me on board, light, with few
>   belongings,
> Almost naked like the children of the sea.
>
> *Antonio Machado*

## Notes

1   Patricia Davis, *Subtle Aromatherapy*. 176.

2   Reiki has a philosophical basis in five simple principles: 'Just for today, do not anger; Just for today, do not worry; We shall count our blessings and honour our fathers and mothers, our teachers and neighbours and honour our food; Make an honest living; Be kind to everything that has life.' From 'The History of Reiki as Told by Mrs Takata', quoted in Diane Stein, *Essential Reiki: A Complete Guide to an Ancient Healing Art*. 26.

# 9
# Creativity in the midst of crisis

To remain vibrant throughout a lifetime we must
always be inventing ourselves, weaving new themes
into our life narratives, remembering our past,
re-visioning our future, re-authorising the myth
by which we live.

*Sam Keen and Anne Valley Fox*

Of all the resources available, time is the most
precious. Use it wisely.

*From 'Bread for the Head'*

The experience of terminal illness turns our lives upside
down and can demand physical, mental and spiritual
resilience, frequently in excess of our ordinary resources
and capacity to cope. There are ways to find peace
and tranquillity, develop awareness, and even experience
a fulfilling joy in the time of dying. For everyone – the
dying person, carers, and family – these can bring much-
needed relief and growth too.

Everyone involved can find an inner healing and wholeness through the process of dying, and facing death. This healing transcends visible circumstances. Frequently the ability to come to terms with loss, grief, despair, anger, guilt, fear and the actual transition of death is both mysterious and astounding. People differ, of course, in their backgrounds and beliefs. Hold lightly to your personal attitudes in the company of others and especially with the dying person. Then everyone can be heard and responded to in their own spiritual terms.

Whatever your views of life and death, these are some practices that can enhance your spiritual life in the terminal phase.

**Meditation**

Meditation is a way to find tranquillity and solace. Through serious, sustained, quiet contemplation, the frenetic outer layers of the mind and emotions are moved aside, creating an inner place of stillness that is quiet and receptive. For believers, the stillness heightens awareness of God; this can be a preparation for true prayer, a dialogue where the mind is more energetically engaged. For others, the quiet state opens up the depths of human consciousness.

We give ourselves a great gift when we shake loose the distractions, noise and clutter that fragment us. Many ordinary people meditate every day. This practice helps ground them in a sphere where time and other concerns don't matter, and where they are not limited by physical constraints.

Science has proved the beneficial effects of a mind brought to stillness and released from anxiety. The simple process of entering the meditative state is deeply relaxing. As physical tension is released, so pain can be alleviated to some extent. Awareness of the breath moving in, through and out of the body is also part of the meditative process and can relieve distress. Some therapists highlight breath-work as a source of healing in itself.

### A special benefit for the dying

The ill person at the last stage of physical life is bedridden and at rest far more than up and about. It's not possible to entertain a sick person all the time, and the dying often find company debilitating and choose solitude. To make matters worse, the ability to read is often impaired. Aimless staring at the wall or picking at night attire and bedclothes can result. (Note: This activity may be caused by opioid overdose. If this is a possibility, consult your health care professional.)

A lot of mental argument and negative thinking creep in with not being able to move and being on one's own. This may result in boredom and depression. Meditation is a great antidote to restlessness, filling the vacuum gently and peacefully.

A caution: Meditation is not meant to replace medication. For anyone new to meditation, it is actually *unwise* to cut back on medicines.

### Getting into meditation

Do try meditating if you haven't done so yet. There are tapes of guided meditations, many books on the subject within the different religious traditions, and several reputable teachers. Suitably contemplative music is freely available. Ask around. Meanwhile, we offer a few guidelines by way of introduction.

The place of meditation needs to be quiet. The ill person should lie or sit well supported and as comfortably as possible; the normal way for others is to sit upright cross-legged in the lotus position, or upright in a chair for those who struggle to sit on the floor. But physical posture is not important – it's the journey within that matters, with its benefit and focus. A period of meditation can last up to 30 minutes or longer, depending on the strength and health of the person.

Here is a simple example of what you can do, with an exercise taking you mentally through your body and into a garden. Through your guided imagination you will start to build up tranquil impressions that focus your attention and thereby calm your mind.

Breathe as well as you can – a little more deeply, slowly, quietly, gently, without strain and effort. Listen to the quiet rhythm of your breath in and out, and close your eyes. Shift your attention gently to your feet, consciously being there and relaxing first the toes, then the rest of the feet and ankles. Progress slowly up the legs, relaxing any tension there. Relax your knees and thighs, including the groin area.

If your mind starts to wander or chatter, gently bring your focus back to the part of the body you were working on. Breathe softly, getting the rhythm back. Some traditions refer to our distractions as 'monkey mind', chattering, scratching, leaping from branch to branch. Note the distraction and return to a place of quiet.

Move up to the whole buttock area, the pelvis and lower abdomen, relaxing all the muscles slowly. Go on to the lower back and up the trunk of the body – consciously relaxing the belly button. The diaphragm should relax. Moving on, relax the back, chest, shoulders, and heart and lungs (by slow, deep, rhythmical breathing). From there go on to the fingers, hands and wrists, lower and upper arms, relaxing the shoulders again, then the neck, jaw, tongue, face, eyes, scalp and whole head.

By completing this part, the active mind is calmed. Consciousness is slowly withdrawn from the outer world to the inner one of stillness and meditation.

Move into a sunlit garden. Visualise its beauty – every detail. At the bottom of this garden is a stream of gurgling crystal sparkling water. Listen to its sound as it moves along. See the sunlight catching on the water and listen to the sounds in this springtime garden – the birds, the bees, the insects, a breeze through the leaves.

Kneel down at the water's edge, cup your hands, taking up the sparkling cool water, and drink it and splash it all over your face. It is refreshing. Bask in the warmth of the golden sun, be at peace, and listen. Allow your whole inner being to be healed in this perfect space of rest.

Breathe more consciously to bring yourself back from this deep place of inner awareness. Slowly and deliberately see your body as filled with radiant light. Think right down into your toes and fingers, open your eyes and have a good stretch. Be at peace. If you have fallen asleep while relaxing, that's fine. Try again later.

## Other sources of comfort and support

### Contemplative thinking

Everyone can expand their consciousness and find peace in contemplation. An effective way to focus and soothe your mind is to take a flower, hold it, and focus on the intricate beauty of the petals, leaves and stem. Feel the texture and reflect on the colours of the petals, while savouring any fragrance. Contemplate the creation of such beauty. You can also dwell on a memory, recalling a special moment in your life when you felt wondrously alive and vital – a time of growth, change and joy.

It is also very fulfilling to dwell on words of wisdom. Carers will cater for what the dying want to hear, which may well be different from what the carers need for themselves: now is the time when we take up the challenge and expand ourselves beyond the limits of our own personal religious identities. The appendix at the end of this book includes verses from the Bible, the Koran, the Torah and other writings that, in our experience, have proved inspirational.

## Music

The human voice in song or chant and the playing of musical instruments are normally helpful as people make the transition into death. We know people who have sung to their loved ones in the moment of dying. Rhythm, tone and melody have a profound effect on the heartbeat, breathing, and the anxious mind. They are calming and releasing, as people have known for centuries – a thousand years ago, for example, the Benedictine monastery at Cluny recorded how monks used music for the dying.

The deep relaxation alleviates the distress of physical or emotional pain if they occur. Often the dying person is weak and possibly in a comatose state as transition approaches, and should not be expending energy on keeping connected with the physical world. The purpose of music now is to help the person move towards completion, aiding in unbinding them from things that could impede a passage of tranquillity. There is an excellent video, *The Chalice of Repose*, on the work of music thanatologists (researchers on death and dying) produced in Canada, which demonstrates these principles.

It is vital that the music suits the person. This is an individual and cultural choice. We have found these helpful for many people: Gregorian chants and the Mass of Angels;[1] two CDs – *Gifts of the Archangels* and *Music Sampler* – by Michael Hammer; recordings of birdcalls, harps and bells; ballads and popular religious songs or hymns sung solo or with full choir; and lullabies, with their soothing nature, particularly for children. For Buddhists, chanting brings peace. African traditions include drums, marimbas, chanting, ululating and song. Islam includes the reciting of sacred texts. Most music stores have a wide range of beautiful recordings that foster tranquillity and contemplation.

There is a difference between music for the living – designed to engage us – and for the dying, which aims to assist people in letting go. The patient's favourite music while they were up and lively is not always that helpful. Of course, it might be what they want even on their deathbed, in which case that is what they should have. Whatever the stage, the patients will know what suits them. Peter says: 'I can remember playing a CD of some jazz music to a young person on her birthday a few weeks before her death. It was a moment beyond compare.'

*Poetry and creative writing*

When a patient is feeling helpless, hopeless and useless, ways of communication are limited. We talk all the time in conversation, of course; but in poetry or other literature words can often be more uplifting because they are so richly used. They can lead people to new discoveries within themselves.

Among other things, poetry can help to heal the fragmented mind, invite stillness in prayer and meditation, and renew appreciation of life by viewing it in another way. The range is vast – through the literature of the ages – and profound. Reflecting on what the religious, philosophical and other writers say aids memory and wise response in a stage of life that is often confusing. Even modest writing can bring comfort, as when children bring poems of their own to sick relatives.

Writing poetry is valuable too. A friend of ours wrote his first poem at the age of eleven as a way of dealing with the grief around his father's death. There is a potential artist in everyone. Where some are more comfortable with drawing or painting to release buried emotion, others may find creative expression in writing a phrase or image that releases pent-up feelings not otherwise easily recognised.

The words said or written when a person is dying are incredibly powerful. They are remembered and quoted by the bereaved long after the death. These words can bless, celebrate and affirm, or have the potential to wound and hurt. They must be chosen with care.

Some social workers working with parents dying from Aids-related illnesses encourage them to fill 'memory boxes' with their own written texts and mementoes so that when the children are older they have something to treasure that expresses the essential spirit and heart of their parents.

Brian, a dying patient who was a keen conservationist, penned specific words to be put on a bench that he wanted erected at a special viewing site on a stretch of Cape coast that he loved. This was done in his memory.

We remember the son of a dying woman writing a poem to his mother in words that were simple, yet powerfully expressive and loving. Poetry can become a coded language expressing gratitude and sadness in a way that transcends the confines of illness. It can be a living link with all who have ever struggled to find meaning in their experience. In a strange way, the very intensity of the suffering can generate the power of transformation, and this is what poetry can express. Read it, and risk writing it too!

### Journals

There is value in keeping a journal during this time of inner struggle and reflection. (Significantly, 'journey' comes from the same root word.) An exercise book next to the bed, for the patient, can track the experience as it happens. Recording developments on the spot can be a relief, and can boost awareness of what is going on. The carer may choose to keep a journal too.

The writing could include scribbled thoughts and images as they arise, or fragments from a dream the night before. All these things help to note the path travelled at a time when much is unclear. They can remind people of their encounters with moments of truth and real inner contentment. Different pen colours could help with the range of what is said. The notes can just be short sentences or phrases, and spelling and grammar don't matter – this is a purely personal record.

If a journal was kept, the dying person may not want to have others reading it. Carers should check the point. If the person chooses to keep the contents private, the book must be burnt unopened. But if there is no objection, the log could become a treasure for family and friends after the death, when there is such a feeling of emptiness and disconnection.

Any personal records can become precious. We heard of a young woman who kept a journal of her travels in Europe. She was hardly home when she was diagnosed with leukemia and died shortly afterwards. Her parents used her journal as a map guide, tracing her route through Europe as a way of mourning her death.

## Sand play

Some people find solace by silently working in a sand tray. This is like using a small Zen Garden tray. You choose objects that suggest themselves to you and put them in the sand. The unconscious mind is freed to access and identify hidden feelings without verbal expression. The therapist guiding the exploration helps the person to access the wisdom of their own inner being.

## Drawing and painting

The use of colour and shape with paints, pastels, and charcoal or lead pencil expresses feelings that are buried or can't be uttered for some reason. Feeling that you can't draw need not be a handicap – this is about expressing, not impressing. Martha, when dying, gleaned comfort from the simple use of finger paints. The adults and children gathered around her using colours to express their emotions.

There is a whole field of study in the relationship we have to colour, and what the colours link to in our mood and deeply rooted feelings. For a full-on basic exercise in colour you need a set of primary colour finger paints, sheets of plain or coloured poster paper, an old shirt or apron, and enough newspaper to protect the large work surface. Play the music that suits the current mood, spread out and mix the paints. Proceed from there, letting creativity take the lead – get your hands and feet involved in the painting process, not trying to produce a masterpiece but expressing your deep emotions with colour, strokes and blobs.

There are times when it's good just to let go and indulge in having fun and messing.

Strong emotions may often surface during this exercise, particularly anger or deep sadness. Tears may appear – let them flow and drip all over the artwork. Afterwards the sense of release of inner pain is a great deal of comfort.

If it is physically possible and the desire is there, consider joining a beginners' art class with a suitably compassionate teacher. For those already versed in drawing and painting, use this time to allow those emotions to express themselves in the most creative way. The results are often surprising.

## Relaxations

Many simple activities help to keep people in focus and prevent boredom and listlessness. They contribute to personal worth, wellbeing and creativity. Patterns, where they are needed, have to be quite easy to do. If the project is too complex, the motivation to do anything might wane. Here are some suggestions, depending on people's ability and physical condition.

### *Handcrafts*

Embroidery, tapestry and other crafts are good diversions from boredom. Even if the work is not completed, this type of activity occupies the hands and can be picked up or left at any time. An occupational therapist working with HIV/Aids patients in Cape Town reports on the patients' delight as they contemplate their creations – special cards, mirrors with mosaic edges, beadwork.

### Puzzles

Interesting jigsaw puzzles on a tray that can be moved around with ease are another way of passing quiet time for the carer, the patient, and children. Crossword puzzles and other word challenges can bring pleasure to some.

### Games

On 'good days', when the spirit is brighter and interest in the surroundings is more attentive, the family could play cards, Monopoly or other board games that lighten the atmosphere and bring in some laughter. Games are a triumph, enabling people to play together despite the confines that illness places on the patient. Participation in this type of light activity helps the patient to still feel part of the immediate family and surroundings, which is particularly important as terminal illness can be so isolating.

A word of caution: Stay on the alert for signs of exhaustion and be sensitive to the patient if there is a desire to stop.

*Being read to*

Many have enjoyed the company and comfort of being read to, and this should be kept up as much as possible. Otherwise, taped books occupy the mind even for short periods. Where our attention span is limited, this is a most welcome aid. A good variety of well-written books, both fiction and non-fiction, has been recorded onto CDs and tapes usable in a standard tape deck. These are available from many bookshops, some libraries, and Tape Aids for the Blind. The Internet is also helpful – amazon.com, exclusivebooks.com and onlineshopping. co.za have a wide range. Borrow from friends and family too.

**The giving of gifts**

Some people at the end of their lives enjoy giving away special items to family members and friends. They have the satisfaction of giving pleasure to others while they are still there. Rini recorded in her journal, 'I feel a lightness each time I give something away – the dress I never wore, the book I loved.'

**Note**

1 '*Adoro te devote*' or, more correctly, '*Adoro devote*', a Eucharistic hymn attributed to St Thomas Aquinas. The common English translation is 'Thee we adore, O hidden Saviour'.

# 10
# Food and nutrition

Food may lose its flavour, but the ritual of sharing
a meal is a celebration of life and a bridge for the
living to remain connected to the dying.

*Peter Fox*

What tantalising morsel of wholesome food
    can I offer
When there is no appetite?
Then there are the cravings
That come and go and move about,
That must be instantly sated
And leave us both exhausted and confused.
Sometimes I wish that my love could nourish you,
Where no food can.

*Sue Wood*

Of all the challenges facing the dying, the family and the
carers, food has the potential to cause the most frustration and distress. Often these reactions are born of ig-

norance and inexperience. Food now is primarily to ease discomfort as people move towards death. This tends to exclude the usual idea of eating to restore or maintain health.

We need to understand that through all the changes brought on by the illness along with the side-effects of aggressive medication, the desire for food in the dying is vastly different from the healthy person's idea of what it should be. Odd cravings appear and appetite in general is diminished.

Most people are very liverish and as a result are highly sensitive to fatty substances and smells, to the point of vomiting and retching. Another factor is deep, all-consuming exhaustion. People are then not able to feed themselves, are even too tired to be fed much, and thus starvation sets in.

Where people have cancer, more often than not the delicate mucous membrane linings of the mouth and digestive tract have been weakened or destroyed by chemotherapy, leaving among other things a very sensitive and at times ulcerated mouth which is dry most of the time. The loss of taste and smell is yet another blow that can upset upset the patient.

Terminally ill people frequently have normal meals placed in front of them, in quantities that take a lot of energy to consume. On the plate, more often than not, are overcooked and very smelly broccoli and flatulence-causing foods – prompting revulsion. It is very difficult for the carers not to be offended when they have lovingly prepared all sorts of tasty morsels to try to tempt the dying person to eat, only to have the food listlessly pushed away, The dying become irritable at attempts to coerce them to eat, and so the spiral descends into hurt and anger on both sides.

A logical solution is to stop trying to provide food that is seen as good and right, and listen to the patient's needs instead. One should jettison the urge to keep the patient eating. Our experience has led to some ideas, given below, that are usually well received by the ill person. Some of the foods mentioned are seasonal and will not be an option at certain times of year. There is, however, enough variety to carry on with.

Spices and seasonings are not appropriate, as these burn the dry mouth. The food needs to be fairly bland. In some instances where taste and smell are impaired, however, full-bodied flavours may be wanted. Here, as usual, personal preference must take the lead. So ask first – or have condiments available on the side to spice up the meal. It's easier to add flavour to a dish than to remove it.

Baby food works well, as it is so easy to digest and very nourishing. Popular choices are apple, pear, butternut and sweet potato. Baby cereal and porridge are well tolerated at times.

Fresh vegetables such as gem squash, mashed potato,

butternut, pumpkin, sweet potato, beetroot, marrows and grated carrots are suitable.

Fresh fruits such as watermelon, sweet melon (*spaanspek*), winter melon, globe melon, seedless white and red grapes, pears, grated apple, paw-paw, papino and fibreless mango are gentle on the digestive tract. Paw-paw and papinos are the best for ulcerated mouths.

Soups, well liquidised, can be served hot or chilled. Popular ones include leek and potato, butternut (no spicy additives like ginger), chicken and vegetable, beetroot and carrot. We found that if the soup was too thick and heavy it was not well received.

As the food needs to be tasty but usually quite bland, colour can sometimes stimulate the waning appetite. Putting different coloured foods on an attractive plate might sometimes work better than having a dull monotone.

Small portions are easier for the patient to cope with, and more attractive.

The best booster is a powdered full-food supplement mixed with water. There are various brands, to be found in most supermarkets. They come in three flavours: chocolate, vanilla and strawberry. Freshly prepared morning and afternoon as a 'shake' in a glass or cup, they give the ailing body enough nutrition for the day. A hinged drinking-straw makes for easy consumption

Ask the health care professional about extra protein

and electrolyte supplements if you need to add nourishment to the diet, particularly if ordinary food becomes difficult to eat or digest. They are available from a dietician, probably in your local chemist or health store.

The following foods may be unsuitable. Some are heavy to digest. But of course, individual tastes are important and a lot depends on how the patient is feeling. This is just a guide, not a rule.

- Heavy fatty foods, creamy sauces, meat in general
- Acidic fruits and vegetables: tomatoes, strawberries, pineapples, oranges, grapefruit, guavas, Kiwi fruit, apricots, bananas (difficult to digest and high in potassium, which is contra-indicated for kidney problems)
- Peppers and egg plant (brinjal) (difficult to digest, and may provoke an allergic reaction)
- Cabbage, broccoli, cauliflower, lentils, beans and pasta (may cause flatulence and provoke distension and discomfort).

With advanced cancer, the abdomen can be distended by secondary tumours in and around the liver, kidneys and stomach. This limits the space for the stomach to expand with food, which is why patients find it easier to eat a little at a time. The lungs are also affected, very often, which tends to result in difficult and shallow breathing. Care should be taken to avoid the patient choking on food and liquids.

When exhaustion takes over, gentle assistance in feeding helps. This is something that busy nursing staff do not always have the time to do in hospitals or Hospices, so feeding is a vital function for family and carers. It takes patience and sensitivity, as the dying so often feel their dignity is compromised. You can encourage a little intake without trying to force the patient to eat (which may cause stress and anxiety). Be guided by the person you are feeding, and you should be able to know roughly when to stop.

Juicing vegetables is a good way of getting nourishment into the body. Carrot, celery and apple make a tasty combination, along with beetroot and apple, cucumber, celery and parsley, and potato juice. Good juicers are available in big stores and are relatively inexpensive.

Diluted fruit juice such as apple, grape, mango or paw-paw is usually appreciated. Again, it is important to steer clear of all acidic fruit and flatulence-causing vegetables – but even this is not a hard-and-fast rule: on a 'good' day, requests for all sorts of things will surprise you. Often people want a glass of sparkling wine or another favourite tipple – give it.

Keep a flask of iced water (with 10 drops of Rescue Remedy added) at the bedside for frequent sipping, as this can relieve a sore mouth. Be guided by the doctors, as some conditions require a controlled intake of fluids. If this is the case, sucking on ice cubes is helpful.

The side-effects of the many drugs administered affect the digestion, and morphine causes constipation, hence the need for very gentle nourishment. Vomiting can happen, sometimes frequently, so dehydration becomes a factor. As death approaches, the need for food falls away and supplemented feeding by a naso-gastric feeding-tube or intravenous drip is stopped. Here, be guided by the professional staff. They are also there to assist carers like yourself.

# 11
# To be read after I am gone

Let us remove death's strangeness; let us practise it;
let us accustom ourselves to it . . . It is uncertain
where death awaits; let us await it everywhere. We
must always be booted and ready to go, as far as it
is in our power. To be ready to die frees us from all
bondage and thraldom.

*Michel Eyquem de Montaigne, Essays*

A widow shared her frustrating story. 'Barnabas has left
such a mess – I can't make head or tail of the insurance
policies or his annuity. I'm getting accounts and I don't
know if he paid them. There are even problems about the
will.' If only she could have said, 'Barnabas was so caring.
Do you know, he even left a file labelled "To be read after
I have gone". In it was his will, the name and phone
number for the insurance company and his funeral poli-
cy. He even left a note on what music he wanted played
at his funeral.'

The time to start the file is now. As an act of love, put all your affairs in order so that they do not cause any anxiety after your death.

**Your Will**

When there is no up-to-date last will and testament, surviving relatives can face problems. They could also be distressed if there is no clarity about your final wishes. Seek advice from an attorney or a legal aid office, and draw up a will to cover all the matters you need to settle. Sign the will, and have it witnessed and kept in a safe place.

If you go to an attorney, choose one who will protect you from unscrupulous fortune hunters, reducing the possibility of manipulation and squabbling out of greed. This situation arises more frequently than one would care to believe.

Banks can also help you make a will. There is an initial fee for drawing it up, and an annual fee for safekeeping and any changes that need to be made.

Choose your executor – one or more, male or female – with care, to ensure that your wishes will be respected. Note that your executor can also be a person who will inherit from your estate.

Do not fear that not having a will means that all assets go to the state. The Law of Intestate Succession ensures that the immediate blood relatives will share the estate after the Master of the High Court has appointed an executor. But remember, dying without a signed will causes long delays in wrapping up the estate.

You must alter your will if circumstances change – beneficiaries may die, marriages dissolve and remarriages occur, and so on.

## Your insurances

Have insurance policies checked, ascertaining existing balances and outstanding loans if any, and keep them together in a safe place with your will.

An important point: Consult an insurance broker or your attorney, or the insurance firm itself, on exactly what you must do to ensure that your spouse or partner receives their full benefit from your retirement annuities – these do not automatically fall under the estate. Get and sign the correct forms. Without this, there is a distinct possibility that all benefits will revert to the insurance firm. It is wise to consult someone with a good name, whom you can trust – to clarify the issue, and complete the paperwork as soon as possible.

Your file should include a list of accounts on which monies are owed, a note of any IOUs or acknowledgements of debt, details of your credit cards and bank or building society accounts, full information on your investments, and so on. Add in the passwords or numbers for such things as cell phones, computers, alarm systems, and cash cards.

Put the file together with your will and other important documents for safekeeping. Tell one or two trusted people where they are held. Do not leave any of this lying around. You could put it all into safe deposit at a bank, or with your attorney, or put it into your safe at home if you have one. Another option is to lock it in a cupboard with your other valuables.

If you are the only parent of under-age or retarded children, or if there are problems with custodianship of these children, you will need to consider very carefully whom you should appoint as legal guardians, to ensure their safety, good nurture and wellbeing. It is wise to seek legal guidance on the matter.

If you live alone, arrange that your pets, if any, are catered for – leave clear instructions for their care and wellbeing.

**Unfinished business**

It seems so cruel that on top of having to deal with the news of our dying, there is another bugbear at the back of our minds – unfinished business. This could be anything from tasks not completed in and around the house, and holidays planned and having to be cancelled, to your relationship with family members, lovers, friends, and business associates. All these things need attention and closure. They could include healing personal rifts.

Really important things left undone create distress and

anger. It is not only the dying who have to be alert and take the initiative. We have seen people dying who have gone without food or water for days on end, holding on for a word or visit from someone important to them, for something to be said, or a message to be given or received.

One of the profoundest tasks for the dying is to come to peaceful terms with themselves. Forgiveness of the self at this coalface is the real balm, not necessarily the faith or lack thereof in a deity. Our basic inner knowledge of the difference between good and bad prods us to consider this huge issue when facing impending death.

The song 'No Regrets' that Edith Piaff sings is wonderful to listen to, but in reality we are often laden with regrets. They have a way of coming to the surface quickly when our time is running out. Those who die suddenly or tragically have no way of addressing these realities. The emotional work is then left to those behind. Saying it like it is can be so helpful at this time – no more covering up, deceit or caution.

We were moved by Thomas's story of how he eliminated his regrets. He raged against the news that he was dying, and at his body, the doctors and God for betraying him. He had a new girlfriend; their relationship was just getting really settled, and he loved her. He also had unfinished business with his ex-wife, and he wanted to be free to love for what time was left.

He phoned an old and trusted friend for help. They talked through the afternoon and well into the early hours of the next morning. Then Thomas called his ex-wife, who came over. Their interaction was frosty. Harsh words were said, but truth was spoken and they apologised to each other for the mess they had made of their life together. They realised the damage their anger and bitterness towards each other had done to their children.

Thomas sat with his children and apologised for his selfishness, and the way things had turned out.

A miracle happened. His children affirmed that they loved and respected him. To them he was the best dad – something he never knew. His rage began to die out. We were not surprised. People need to be told how special they are. It is important not to leave eulogies until after they have gone, in a death notice in the local paper or during the service. These sentiments are so valuable and constructive when expressed appropriately to the person while alive.

Thomas had one more thing to do. He phoned his old and trusted friend again. She came to him. He told her how much he loved her, and had done ever since their brief affair ten years earlier. He'd hoped they would get together, but watched her walk away into the arms of the man she loved. She was still his best friend.

This set Thomas free. He had happiness and the love he sought with his new girlfriend. They shared eight months of life together before he died in peace.

**Planning the funeral or memorial ceremony**

Some people, when they are seriously ill, like to say clearly what they want for the ritual after their death. Others choose not to discuss such matters, or simply trust the instincts of those organising the event.

Leave any instructions about your funeral or memorial ceremony with your will, for safekeeping. Even healthy people should do this now – it makes life much easier if anything happens resulting in sudden death. Then others will know they are making arrangements in accordance with the deceased's wishes. (Hospice also tries to cater for what people would like. If they are atheist or agnostic, this is respected in the ceremony arranged for them.)

The range of rituals around death and mourning offer practical comfort and support. Often the religious ones facilitate a connection to a higher being and enable the bereaved to sense the meaning and value of the life that has been lived.

A ritual event is an opportunity for closure and farewell. It is clearly an emotional experience and one that requires emotional honesty. It is helpful to all concerned for the person who is dying to give clear instructions as to what they want in the ceremony and how they would like it to be conducted.

Has the patient requested burial or cremation? Sometimes very specific feelings are attached to the choice. Talking frankly about this is helpful all round.

A ritual such as a funeral gives those who are grieving an opportunity to focus on memories of their loved one. This is comforting in the face of huge loss and the subsequent feeling of emptiness. The loving way in which family and friends come together at a funeral creates a new sense of solidarity among the living. Facing death gives them a perspective on the real meaning of life. There is a moving away from pettiness and saying hurtful things, and realisation that our life span is short.

All this is important for closure. Such an event also marks that the threshold has been crossed, where a new chapter begins for everyone. This does not mean that the bereaved put things behind them at once, of course. The real work of grief management and bereavement begins once the funeral is over.

If family members arrive from different parts and have not seen the deceased person, it may be important for them to view the body and make their farewells. If the process of dying has been prolonged and difficult, there is little need for a final viewing of the body by those who accompanied it in the last stages of its journey.

Simple rituals at the ceremony help the grieving process – lighting candles, displaying a photograph. Including something of the deceased's that indicates where their heart lay – a walking stick, a well-loved hat – gives a personal touch that aids an emotional connection.

A collage of pictures reflecting the life of the person also helps to evoke the life being remembered.

The ceremony is the place for honest leave-taking, and not to eulogise or idealise the one who died. We suggest an honest reflection on the pros and cons of the person's life to show what was complete and whole and what was broken and unfinished.

Some people want their ceremony, when they die, to be a celebration too. A wake or a get-together with food and drink could be an important part of being remembered. In some cultures this is an essential part of the death ritual. In others, it could be irreverent and inappropriate.

Rituals vary greatly. In Xhosa tradition, at least a week of evening prayers for the family and neighbours should precede the funeral. The Muslim requirement is very different, requiring burial before sunset on the day of death. Whatever the cultural and religious customs, they are there to assist the emotions at a time of grief and loss.

If the dying person is able to speak quite plainly about their ritual, this is surely a sign of the relinquishment that a good preparation for death requires of us.

# 12
## Palliative care

Pain is not a simple sensation like seeing or hearing; it is far more complex. Aristotle described it as a 'passion of the soul'. It certainly reflects a major area of body–mind interaction.

*Robert Twycross and Sylvia Lack*

Palliative care is defined as the total care of people with far advanced, progressive illness, with a diminishing life expectancy. Active treatment is no longer an option.

To the casual observer, palliative care is pain and symptom control. But it also has a role to play in freeing the patient from unnecessary, undignified suffering.

Palliative care, according to the World Health Organisation:

- Provides relief from pain and other distressing symptoms
- Affirms life and regards dying as a normal process
- Intends neither to hasten nor postpone death

- Integrates the psychological and spiritual aspects of patient care
- Offers a support system to help patients live as actively as possible until death
- Offers a support system to help the family cope during the patient's illness and in their own bereavement
- Uses a team approach to address the needs of patients and their families, including bereavement counselling, if indicated
- Will enhance quality of life, and may also positively influence the course of illness
- Is applicable early in the course of illness, in conjunction with other therapies that are intended to prolong life, such as chemotherapy or radiation therapy, and includes those investigations needed to better understand and manage distressing clinical complications.

**Morphine**

We wish to dispel any myths about morphine. Sometimes people equate the word with being at the end of the road, and so they avoid this stronger painkiller. The use of properly titrated morphine in correctly prescribed dosage has, however, played a significant role in the successful management of pain. Medical supervision is essential. Sometimes patients try to set their own medication routines, which can have disastrous consequences.

Like codeine, morphine eases pain and discomfort by acting on the pain centres in the brain and spinal cord. Morphine is used to control pain that no longer responds to codeine or similar drugs. It is used at many different stages of the illness – not just at the end. The dosage is carefully increased or decreased as necessary and is given at set times, usually during the day and at night. The liquid suspension can be mixed with fruit juice or milk to mask its bitter taste.

The main unwanted side-effects include constipation, vomiting, drowsiness, nausea, unsteadiness and disorientation. These side-effects are all treatable. If the drug is properly prescribed, administered and supervised, the side-effects are not necessarily that severe. Other side-effects, including sweating and a dry mouth, usually pass, and the mind clears again after the first few days of treatment. Laxatives, fluid intake and dietary fibre all help with bowel function.

Morphine is administered in various forms: liquid suspension, injection, tablets, or via a syringe-driver. The attending doctor can also prescribe analgesic skin patches that are effective and easy to apply.

The syringe-driver is a useful device. Used under qualified supervision, it is available on loan from most Hospices. The rationale of the syringe-driver is to have a pump that intermittently delivers a measured dose of morphine into the bloodstream for continuous pain relief, by means of an intravenous needle set through the skin. This tool restores confidence and dignity, as it is small enough to rest under the bedclothes next to the patient.

## A broader view of pain
Robert Twycross and Sylvia Lack, whom we quoted at the beginning of this chapter, say:[1]

Pain is not a simple sensation like seeing or hearing; it is far more complex. Aristotle described it as a 'passion of the soul'. It certainly reflects a major area of body–mind interaction. Intensity of pain is modified not only by medication but also by mood, morale and the meaning of the pain to us as individuals. Living with [serious illness] is hard work and there are often plenty of negative factors to contend with – loss of energy, loss of job, and financial independence, and so on. All these factors, and more, influence how sensitive we are to any underlying physical pain sensations. We have tried to put these ideas together in the following diagram:

## Factors influencing pain sensitivity

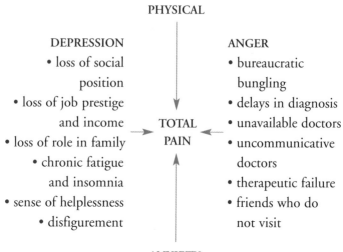

other symptoms
unwanted effects of treatment

PHYSICAL

DEPRESSION
- loss of social position
- loss of job prestige and income
- loss of role in family
- chronic fatigue and insomnia
- sense of helplessness
- disfigurement

TOTAL PAIN

ANGER
- bureaucratic bungling
- delays in diagnosis
- unavailable doctors
- uncommunicative doctors
- therapeutic failure
- friends who do not visit

ANXIETY
- fear of hospital or nursing home
- fear of pain
- worry about family and finances
- fear of death
- spiritual unrest, uncertainty about future

Relaxation, exercises and the use of simple meditation and visualisation assist the patient in easing pain in non-physical terms.

**Being a companion for the dying**

We fully endorse the advice from Cynthia Birrer, of the Pathways Institute of Thanatology, for those who find themselves in the role of carer: 'Those who love the dying help by sitting silently, by listening, by being available to talk, to touch and to share. What we want is to help them achieve what we wish for ourselves – a good death, a *euthanatos*.'[2]

Birrer passes on the invaluable core idea of Dame Cecily Saunders, who helped to pioneer Hospice in Britain, that 'all the needs of the dying are summed up in the words "Watch with me" . . . The word "watch" says many things. It demands that our work with the dying should stem from respect for them and that we pay very close attention to their distress. What the dying person needs is both skill and compassion.'[3]

On what real watching means, Dame Cecily has this to say:

> We have to learn what it feels like to be so ill, to be leaving life and its activity, to know that your faculties are failing, that you are passing from loves and responsibilities. We have to learn how to 'feel with' the dying without 'feeling like' them if we are to give the kind of listening and steady support that they need to find their own way through.

From the caregiver's view, then, what a dying person needs beyond physical care is someone to take him seriously, care about him, listen to him, and get to know him as a person so that he is appreciated as such.

The commonest failing among caregivers is their inability to listen or to deal with what is actually said. The reason is that during a conversation a person with a fatal illness usually says one or more things that make his caregiver nervous and uncomfortable. References to fear, resentment, anger, despair or death make the listener so uneasy that she simply ignores them or literally shuts the person up by saying something like 'Don't talk that way' or 'Don't worry, you'll be O.K.'

We say 'How are you?' to our friends but always with the tacit understanding that under no circumstances will they say anything but 'Fine'.

What does one talk about with a person who is fatally ill? Too often we forget that the dying person is a living person. He has both a past and a present history, his own talents and idiosyncrasies, his unique interests and viewpoints. Basically one goes to talk with a dying person for the same reason one goes to talk with a living person: because of an interest in him. Dealing with him should be viewed as getting to know him better.

Talk about those things that make the person more real to you – his family, his work, his current interests, his loves and hates, particularly as they affect him now, but with care to include his past and present.[4]

Communication with the dying does not have to be verbal. There are many other ways to convey love and concern: the gentle squeeze of a hand, a silence shared or a hug. Touch is one of the most important forms of saying what words fail to do. There have been many occasions where the partner (or parent, in the case of a child) has climbed carefully onto the bed with the dying person and held them gently in their arms. This is one of the most comforting acts that one can do, for both parties.

The dying, particularly those with Aids, have sadly become almost the untouchables of this age. Misunderstanding and ignorance are to blame; but the simple touch on a hand or arm, a hug, or holding a hand or foot is very comforting *and perfectly safe*.

This anonymous overview of what the dying experience and need comes from a notice board at the nurses' station of St Luke's Hospice in Kenilworth, Cape Town:

The process of death confronts us with a diseased body that needs diagnosis and must be able to trust its carers.

The disobedient body, no longer under control, needing to find new areas of independence, competence and strength.

The vulnerable body, consumed by anticipation, needing to be given security and support it can trust.

The violated body, invaded and open to medical scrutiny, needing sensitive help to maintain some dignity.

The enduring body, whose horizons have shrunk through huge discomfort, needing support.

The resigned body that has learned to relinquish its former self and needs assistance to accept and rebuild.

The deceiving body that, with illness, has progressed silently to the point of a late discovery needing reassurance with the appropriate treatment.

The betraying body that breaks down from hidden stress, needing watchful care and assistance to recognise and resolve such problems, and the betraying mind that performs in unusual ways, needing support and encouragement.

# Notes

1   Robert G. Twycross and Sylvia A. Lack, *Oral Morphine: Information for Patients, Families and Friends*. 23.

2   'Wages of Love: The Experience of Loss', handout material from the Symposium of the Pathways Institute of Thanatology held at the University of the Witwatersrand, Johannesburg on 6–7 February 1979.

3   Ibid.

4   Ibid.

# 13
# Practical care at home

Compassion for the sick and dying is easy;
responding with insight, skill and love is the
challenge.

*Sue Wood and Peter Fox*

With the increase in terminal illnesses such as cancer and
HIV/Aids, caring for the dying at home is no longer a
choice. This is true for almost everyone. State hospitals
are an option but they do send some dying patients
home, for lack of staff and resources or ward closures due
to lack of funds. Private nursing homes and frail care
centres in old age homes cater for the frail and dying, if
you can afford the cost. But with those realities, most
people tend to choose home care.

Hospice can help to some extent. Most Hospices with
an in-patient facility will, for a period of time, admit
patients thus:

* up to 14 days to relieve the family

- from 3 to 20 days for symptom control and pain management
- for final-stage terminal care as death approaches.

But home care can work very well indeed. The prospect may be new and daunting, yet caring for the ailing body requires much the same equipment as one uses when caring for babies and young children. Much of what we say here will be familiar.

**The bed**

As frailty increases and more time is spent in bed, it is wise for the patient to be in a single bed to facilitate nursing care. A double bed limits carers to working on one side only, which makes it difficult to lift, move or turn the person safely and comfortably without distress to them and injury to the carers. It helps to have one person on either side to change linen and bedclothes. Remember there may be much discomfort in spite of medication, so any movement needs to be done at the pace of the patient – slowly and carefully.

If you don't have a single bed and can't buy one, ask your willing wider family and friends. If circumstances permit, hiring a hospital bed is a good option as the height is adjustable. Hospital beds are designed to give maximum comfort and address the needs of both the patient and the carer. Hospice can help you source one.

Use extra pillows to support the body. When a patient

is lying on the side, place a pillow between the knees, another between the arms and in front of the stomach area, and one supporting the pelvic area at the back. This comforts and gives a sense of security. When the patient is sitting up and needs to lean forward, a pillow can be put over the abdominal area to support the arms. When the patient is lying back on a wedge, a pillow should be placed under the knees and an egg-box cushion under the heels.

A wedge is the answer to being propped up by pillows that travel and slip and require frequent repositioning. This foam shape has two angles of support, 90 and 45 degrees, depending on the side used. Cover it with a continental pillowcase for protection. You can buy a wedge at any medical supply store or a pharmacy that sells medical equipment. A small pillow can be used behind the neck for comfort; again, the patient is supported at an angle of either 90 or 45 degrees.

Wedges have a pocked 'egg-box' surface and so do some foam mattress covers and small cushions. This finish helps to prevent the pressure sores so common in bedridden patients.

Fitted sheets in all bed sizes, and pillow protectors with a towelling top and a waterproof backing (made under the name Snugfit), are available from most outlets stocking bed linen. The towelling surface reduces sweating. The waterproof backing does not crackle or make a noise as the patient shifts around on the bed. These fitted sheets can also be tumble-dried.

You need adequate bed linen. Borrow extra if necessary. The very ill and frail person in this condition can suffer from profuse periods of sweating, particularly at night. If the weather is cold, it is important to keep the patient warm and dry. Cotton T-shirts help to absorb some of the moisture.

As the skin and body become sensitive, light duvets or rugs provide warmth. The frail body cannot tolerate heavy blankets and duvets. If you do not own anything suitable, borrow from friends or ask Hospice for assistance. Sheepskin is soft and comfortable to lie on and is also particularly useful in the wheelchair. A ring also helps with sitting in bed or in a chair, and protects the buttock area.

If the foot of the bed needs to be raised, proper bed raisers can be loaned from Hospice. Bricks also do a good job. Ensure that both legs are firmly set to prevent them from slipping off the support base.

If possible, move the bed nearer to a window so that the patient can see outside instead of facing a blank wall, This adds quality to days when most of the time is spent in bed, and is a simple thing to do.

### Clothing and useful extras

As the frailty increases, use *tops* that open down the front or back for ease of changing, with the least disturbance to the frail and ailing body.

A *convenience vest* is a clever idea. Take a vest and cut through the shoulder straps at the top. Then join the two cut ends with Velcro, press-studs or a button and button-hole. This makes it very easy to examine the patient and change dressings. Normal night attire can be awkward for breast-cancer patients in particular, when they have drips inserted, need to be examined, or have dressings changed.

You need soft, absorbent *towels* for bed-bathing – the bigger the better – so that the bed linen does not get wet.

A *wheelchair* is invaluable for moving the ill person around the house or for a short break outside when the weather is good. Debilitating weakness calls for this assistance, as the patient often prefers to use the limited energy available for spending time with family. You can hire wheelchairs from medical supply stores. Hospice usually has some available as well.

Always take great care when pushing a wheelchair. It does not enhance the condition of the patient if they find themselves being 'wheelied' round corners. Exercise particular caution when trying to negotiate bumpy, uneven surfaces or steps. Remember, the passenger in the wheelchair is very fragile and often in some discomfort. Unnecessary jarring and tilting causes anxiety and exacerbates pain.

There is a unique and easy-to-operate *hoist* called 'Up

U Go', designed to enable a patient to be lifted off the bed and gently swung across over a wheelchair and then lowered – at the touch of a button. Returning the patient to the bed works in reverse. The patient is securely held by two wide straps. This clever invention is bolted to the wall next to the bed and designed to lift up to 110 kg. (For contact details, see Contacts at the end of this book.)

As time progresses and the body weakens, it is best to have a *commode* next to the bed for toilet use. Bedpans are difficult to use and most uncomfortable. Other options are to consider *catheterisation*, or the use of *adult incontinent pads* or *nappies*. As very little food is being absorbed or digested, most of the waste is urine. The nursing sisters from Hospice will help with these procedures and teach you how to empty the bag and replace it.

**The bathroom**
Bathing in a bath is too energy-sapping. Getting a weak body in and out becomes difficult for the patient and the helper. You can hire a bath 'chair' from a medical equipment outlet or borrow one from Hospice: this useful equipment has a seat that straddles the bath firmly.

If there is a shower, the patient could sit on a plastic garden chair while the helper, wearing a bathing costume or their birthday suit (depending on the relationship), helps with the washing process. Handheld showerheads attached to the taps in the bath work just as well, with a stool well secured in the bath itself.

*Never* leave a patient alone in the bath or shower. There may be sudden attacks of faintness or dizziness. Check the water temperature. It must be warm enough for comfort. Hot water affects blood pressure and can cause dizziness and faintness.

Keep your eyes open as you help the patient along to the shower. Pain control medication can affect perception of the height of steps and many other things.

## Preventing injury to the carer

When caring for someone who is weak or injured and unable to move without aid, there can be a risk of muscle and joint injury. Lower back pain or injury can be caused by a sudden overload – for example, catching a person who faints suddenly – or from repetitive overload like lifting or moving a patient frequently.

We sought advice from a chiropractor, Dr Tim Wood, to help against the risk of injury to both the carer and patient.

### *Moving the patient*

*Never* attempt to lift or move a patient on your own. Work with another carer – that's the first safety rule.

If the area around the bed or chair is cramped, the risk of injury is higher. Your posture could be awkward and your body unbalanced as you try to lift or move your patient. Create enough space to move. This may mean moving side tables or drip stands gently away from both sides of the bed. Make sure that the floor is not slippery. Move loose rugs away from the area where you are working.

Check that your own clothing and that of the patient will not hook onto anything like the arm of a chair. Wear shoes with rubber soles for extra grip. Have both feet firmly on the floor, hip-width apart, and bend the knees slightly to anchor yourself well before lifting the patient.

**Log-rolling.** This technique turns a patient to lie on their side. The manoeuvre is useful when you change bed linen, give a bed-bath or gentle back-rub, or pull down a sliding sheet.

Where possible, at least two people (depending on the size of the patient) should perform this task. Always roll the patient towards yourselves – never away from you. This task must be coordinated so that the carers gently turn the patient all at the same time and pace. Follow these steps:

1. Turn the patient's head gently towards the carers.
2. Gently bend the patient's arm closer to the helper at the elbow, placing it out of the way.
3. Place the further arm across the patient's chest.
4. Cross the far leg over the one nearer the helper.
5. Using the patient's shoulder and knee as levers,

gently *roll* the patient towards you. Another carer standing on the opposite side of the bed ensures that the patient does not roll off the bed.

### Working safely together with the patient's assistance

Most people, even when ill and weak, want to have some form of independence and don't wish to be a burden on others. This is a good thing, as moving is made so much easier for both parties if the patient is able to help.

As long as it is physically possible for the patient to move alone, with a little assistance, encourage this. If you are working as a team and communicating well, the task is not so difficult.

Listen carefully to what the patient intends to do, and work together, ensuring that everyone – the patient and carers – clearly understand what move is going to be made.

Always make the move at the patient's pace, gently and carefully minimising discomfort where you can.

**Helping the patient to sit up in bed.** Always encourage the patient, where possible, to sit up using their own strength. A rope ladder or a knotted rope can be fixed to the end of the bed so that bedbound patients can pull themselves forward, enabling the carer to adjust the wedge or cushions behind them comfortably.

Another way is for carers to stand on either side of the bed. The patient grips the carers at the elbows. Patients then pull themselves up. Once they are sitting up, one helper hugs and holds up the person while the other rearranges the back rest and pillows.

Do not let the patient fall backwards.

**Injury to the patient**
If you, the patient, are injured,

- tell your health care professional the full story and then
- take action on the advice given: do exercises or take medication as prescribed
- complete the course of care agreed upon
- don't miss appointments
- tell the health care professional of any changes in your condition, whether good or bad.

Your voice always needs to be given a fair hearing. There may be times when you will not like accepting the sort of treatment prescribed. If you have a strong objection, discuss it with your health care professional and negotiate a way forward that will suit you and also benefit you medically.

**Injury to the carer**
In spite of taking care, injury sometimes still does occur. These injuries normally affect the back, neck and shoulders. Go for treatment as soon as there any is pain or discomfort. Don't leave an injury of this nature untreated.

There are many therapies to choose from, including massage and physiotherapy (see Chapter 8), and body stress release, chiropractic and acupuncture (Chapter 7). Your health care professional may prescribe an anti-inflammatory to ease the pain.

Whatever kind of therapist you want to consult, these ideas will help you find one who suits your needs:

- Ask friends and family who have had similar problems to recommend someone who helped them.
- The consulting rooms should be fairly close by. (Driving for long periods can be very stressful and it is not ideal after having treatment.)
- Discuss the cost, how often you will need to be seen, and for how long a period.
- Beware of people insisting that you buy masses of 'remedies' or an expensive 'new' device.
- Don't be afraid to get a second opinion.
- Try to look for a practitioner who offers more than just symptom relief.
- If you feel uncomfortable or uneasy about a particular approach or personality – move on.

**How can you avoid problems and speed recovery?**
It's the old story of leading as healthy a lifestyle as possible (mental, emotional, spiritual, as well as physical). The concepts are quite simple and are all about 'What we take in and what we put out'.

'Taking in' refers to diet. Particularly when emotional and mental stress are prevalent, we often increase body stress by not nourishing it with the right foods. Eat a varied diet including plenty of fresh fruit and vegetables, avoid fatty or fried foods, and cut down on salt and preservatives.

'Putting out' refers to the energy expended during physical activity. Regular exercise is good. Aerobic exercise not only benefits the heart, lungs and muscular-skeletal system, but also has an amazing ability to improve our moods and our mental state. Get into a routine. Aerobic exercise should be done three to four times a week. For those who can't do this, swimming and walking are activities available to all.

In addition to the exercises mentioned, you will need to strengthen the areas you use in helping a bedbound patient. 'Core stabilising' is popular at present for lower back problems, with programmes such as Pilates being used more widely. They focus on strengthening the lower back and the tummy muscles (the abs – short for 'abdominals').

If you can afford it, it's a good idea to attend a gym or get a qualified instructor or personal trainer to help you learn how to do these exercises correctly.

There are many stretching and strengthening exercises that can easily be done at home. Pelvic tilts, bend-knee sit-ups, crunches, thigh extensions (kick-backs), and thigh abductors and adductors are just a few of them. The cat stretch and hamstring and gluteus stretches are simple to do and helpful in alleviating and preventing back pain. These need to be done regularly to get the benefit – so get into the routine!

**Nursing the dying body**
Your general equipment should include the following: surgical gloves, aprons, cotton wool, KY jelly, gauze dressings of various sizes, a roll of clingfilm, talcum powder, lanolin-based cream for pressure-sore areas, aqueous cream for general dry skin, disinfectant, and hand-washing soap. Never discard used syringes, needles, used dressings or any other used medical materials into your ordinary dustbin. Special containers for the disposal of hazardous medical waste can be obtained with the help of Hospice, your GP or day care clinic. At the same time, find out whom you should contact to collect the containers.

In the terminal stages the body is often thin, with no muscle-padding on the shoulders, lower back and pelvic area. The skin can become paper-thin. Circulation is poor and pressure sores result. Other areas to watch are the elbows, heels, back of head and ears – all the bony parts on which the body rests either in a sitting or lying position.

In order to prevent pressure sores (also known as bedsores), massage the affected areas gently, using circular motion, with lanolin-based cream every one or two hours during the day and at least twice during the night. Experience shows that a stoma plaster over the coccyx area at the bottom of the spine is helpful in certain cases.

Family members can help with this care. One family we know worked in rotation, choosing suitable times for their turn and also sharing the night massages. This ensured quality and continuous loving care without the burden resting on just one individual.

Though it is important to try to prevent bedsores, consider first the comfort of the patient. As the active illness progresses, moving the patient causes much more discomfort, however gently done. A point will be reached when it is not possible to reduce the disturbance any further.

It is not advisable to insist on moving the patient if this activity is causing very considerable discomfort. There comes a time when it is best to allow the patient to lie quietly, undisturbed and without pain.

# 14
# Final crossing: The last 48 hours

How people die remains in the memories of those
who live on.

*Dame Cecily Saunders*

## The last 48 hours

As you wait alongside and watch the patient, certain signs
may precede death. A few days to a few hours before-
hand, you may notice things like limited attention span
with disorientation, difficulty in swallowing, drowsiness,
and lack of interest in food and liquids. In more detail,
this is what to look for:[1]

## *Metabolism*

Metabolic disturbances may be responsible for changes in
the mental state. These may range from lethargy to
delirium.

- Sleep patterns may change: there may be increased
  daytime sleep, *or* the day and night pattern may be
  reversed.

- There may be difficulty in waking or in effecting responses.
- The person may be disorientated.
- The person may be more restless, picking at bedcovers (this can also stem from opiate medication).
- An increase in anxiety, fear and loneliness at night may occur.
- The patient may go for 3–5 days without any intake of food or water.
- You may notice jerky, uneven, involuntary movements.

**What to do.** Stay calm, speak quietly, use a gentle touch. Discontinue all unnecessary medications. Maintain comfort and symptom control.

### Muscle tone
These signs may distress the bystanders but they are normal and cause no distress to the dying person.
- Expect flaccidity in the extremities.
- There may be involuntary moaning on expiration as the upper airway muscles relax.

### Senses
- Vision may become blurry or dim.
- The person may feel hot (diaphoresis) and not want to be covered.

- Hearing acuity may decrease though it is thought to be last to disappear.

**What to do.** Use indirect lighting. Assume that the patient can hear. Continue to speak directly to the patient, explaining the care they are receiving.

## Respiration
- Breathing becomes uneven in rate and rhythm as the circulation weakens and waste material builds up. This is known as Cheyne-Stoke respiration.
- Breathing may cease (apnoea) for up to a minute or more.
- Secretion in the back of the throat (the posterior pharynx) may rattle. This is commonly called the 'death rattle'.

**What to do.** Reposition the head, raising it and turning it to the side. Put a small fan at the bedside, as oxygen will probably not help the patient at this stage.

## Elimination
- Urine will be darker and decrease in amount.
- Incontinence will probably occur.
- Retention may occur due to enlarged prostate, weakness, lack of awareness, or medications.

**What to do.** Continue to treat constipation as it may cause nausea or vomiting. Maintain good hygiene, protect bedclothes, and ask the attending professional to use a catheter if distension is suspected.

*Secretions*
- These will be thicker due to dehydration.
- They may pool at the back of the throat.
- They may be copious, as in pulmonary oedema.

**What to do.** A humidifier in the room may be helpful. Give the patient small pieces of crushed ice if they can be tolerated. Turn the patient gently onto the left side to facilitate drainage. Note that this stage causes more anxiety for the family than for the semi-comatose or comatose patient.

*Circulation*
- Extremities will become cool.
- Skin of the extremities may become dark or mottled.
- Other areas of the body may become dusky or pale.

**What to do.** Avoid electric blankets. Cover the patient with a clean sheet or other covering of your choice.

**Last services before death**

Lack of interest in fluids and resultant dehydration in a person close to death reduce the need for a bedpan or catheter, and a natural reduction in pulmonary secretions means less congestion and coughing. But small quantities of water administered by syringe or teaspoon help relieve dryness in the mouth. Lip-ice or Vaseline smeared gently on the lips helps soothe cracks.

As death approaches, the patient may tend to slip in and out of consciousness. It is vital that family and other loved ones are called early enough to give them time to travel long distances if necessary and to arrive when the patient is still able to say goodbye.

The dying person may have something of importance to tell you, so watch for signs of attempts at communication.

Goodbyes can be said and constant reassurance given to the dying person. Being with the person, speaking calmly, and gently holding a hand are crucial to facilitating a peaceful departure. At this time it is important to impart words of appreciation and affirmation of the life that has been lived.

Hopelessness and helplessness, if they are felt, can result in acute suffering – hence the need for calm and gentle encouragement. Jiddu Krishnamurti, one of the most revered spiritual teachers, once asked a group of listeners what they would say to a close friend who is about to die. Their answers dealt with assurances, words about beginnings and endings, and various gestures of compassion. He stopped them short. 'There is only one thing you can say to give the deepest comfort. Tell them that in their death a part of you dies and goes with them. Wherever they go, you go also. They will not be alone.'[2]

## At the time of death

The process of death can appear very distressing to those around the bed. Jerks and spasms, noisy breathing and grunting can occur. These are motor functions and do not necessarily indicate that the person is actually suffering. Even so, any bystanders who have the need to be always in control can find the dying process overwhelming.

These things will happen:
- Respiration ceases.
- There may be a sudden emptying of the bladder and bowel.
- Colour becomes ashen or waxy white.
- The pulse stops.
- The jaw relaxes and eyes are fixed.

Sometimes death occurs peacefully while the person is asleep. There are other times when there is a loss of consciousness and a general slowing down of vital signs. This is the time when the family can sit quietly together with their loved one. A trusted relative, partner or caregiver can remove all jewellery. Someone can call the attending doctor and (depending on the religion) the priest, elder, rabbi, imam or other spiritual confidant.

After death has occurred, there may be the ritual cleansing of the body by the appropriate people, and dressing in favourite clothes or night attire. This in many religions has ritual significance but is not always done these days – again, it is a matter of choice. The body just needs to be laid out straight with a pillow under the head as if the deceased were simply peacefully asleep.

At the moment of death there may be discharges from some of the orifices of the body. The body is then cleaned. The clothed body is then laid flat with the arms straight at the side or folded on the chest. Any tubes or needles are removed from the body. Colostomy and urosomy bags are left in place. If there are dentures, they are replaced in the mouth and the eyes are closed. Try to keep the mouth in a closed position by placing a folded towel under the chin. The body is usually removed, not later than six hours after death, by the funeral directors.

Prayers are conducted, depending on the religious beliefs of the family, and the last goodbyes said.

### After the last goodbyes

The doctor, Hospice or family representative will then have to contact the undertakers, who will collect the body after the death certificate has been completed, signed and issued by the attending doctor or sister.

There should be no hurry to have the body removed; treat the room as you would a sacred space, clearing it of clutter. Depending on cultural tradition and beliefs, the lighting of a candle may be appropriate, along with putting flowers in place. A quiet time is soothing here, as family members and friends may move in and out of the room.

Once death has come and gone, the death certificate, which is required along with the will by the Master of the High Court, must be presented to whoever is handling the estate (often a bank or an attorney). The death must be recorded at the Department of Home Affairs with certified copies of the death certificate, the ID of the deceased, and proof of the ID of the person attending to these issues.

Appointing a funeral director is an important task. There are affordable ones. It is wise to get several quotes first, and find out exactly what the firms require and offer. Choose someone the family feel is appropriate. You will also need to decide about burial or cremation, and the final resting-place. Some cemeteries and memorial parks have 24-hour security, lighting from dusk to dawn, and other facilities. Such places may be preferred by people who want good grave maintenance and safe access to the site. These discussions usually happen before the event of death, and are guided by the dying person's wishes.

It is wise to choose a family representative to make all those difficult but necessary telephone calls on their behalf, giving news of the death and making arrangements, bearing in mind that sensitivity is needed. Often the spouse or partner, son or daughter, or perhaps a good friend may volunteer. It is not an easy task, as the process of grieving may well have begun. Having to break the news to others involves being exposed to their shock, sorrow and distress. No matter how much the approaching death of a person may have been anticipated and even accepted, the actual happening can still be heartbreaking. The apparent finality of it all creates shock too.

This is a busy time, as family, colleagues and loved ones pour in to support the closely bereaved. The day of the funeral or memorial service comes and goes, and life returns to normal for those on the periphery. All those who rallied round go back to their busy lives, and those who were very close begin the process of bereavement and adjustment, reconstituting a life without the companionship of the departed. Day-to-day chores have to be attended to, the business of life has to go on. This can help people to cope too.

Those whose lives have quickly returned to normal still have a role to play. Sending a simply worded note, a loving phone call, a bunch of flowers (if appropriate culturally), an offer of assistance or a meal goes a very long way to lifting and healing the feeling of aloneness and isolation. It is well to remember that when people are bereaved they are like a bird with a broken wing – unable to fly until time mends the break. They need gentle loving support to help them prepare for their return into the world's mainstream of business and insensitivity. For the longer term, diarising a few anniversary dates is a very kind and compassionate act too.

Bereavement- and grief-counselling are invaluable in aiding the mourning folk to re-enter the mainstream of life once more. Everyone close to the death – partners, carers, children, whoever they are – feels more or less exhausted in body, mind and spirit. They need periods of comfort, rest and perhaps solitude.

Practical things take time. The distribution of personal effects, particularly clothing, may be almost impossible to do at first. Rushing into things may not be beneficial. Take time.

Wearing an item of the deceased's clothing can be very comforting. Grieving people tell us this brings much-needed relief for 'that bruised and broken feeling'.

## Note

1   The following section to the bottom of page 155 is quoted directly with permission from a handout entitled 'The Last 48 Hours' issued by the Ohio Hospice and Palliative Care Organization, Ohio, and the Hospice of Lancaster County, Pennsylvania, United States.

2   Quoted in Frederick and Mary Anne Brussat (ed), *Spiritual Literacy: Reading the Sacred in Everyday Life*. 404.

# 15
## Sunset: Last reflections

May your life upon earth become as a dream to
your waking soul and may your thirsting eyes
behold a glorious new sunrise beyond the
denseness of the earth.

*From the Sufi Prayer for the Dead*

Dying alive is a journey we all embark on. Clear channels
of communication help us deal with our distress. Often,
however, our human condition of pride, anger and stubbornness prevents clarity. How can we ease this passage?
It is always a journey without certainty. Such a journey
into the unknown can be one of growth, peace and
understanding. It can also be a frightening experience.
We make the choice. This book is written in the hope
that it will equip the dying for the choices they must
make, and everyone for the creative roles they can play.
The transition from this life to the next, we authors
believe, can be a profound and conscious experience, a
celebration of life.

The living connections that have sustained us in life shift as the dying process begins. These connections are changed – not lost. Saying goodbye to our own life and to those who love us is the hardest assignment for any human being. But we, even dying, are more powerful than we can imagine. The resources within our own inner life and the caring community around us give this journey a safer context.

For those who are dying, and also for ourselves after their death, it is vitally important that we affirm people's qualities and tell them what we love and admire in them while they are alive. And of course, we shouldn't wait until people are on their deathbeds for this, but make it our regular practice.

No matter how well prepared everyone may be, the actual event of parting still comes as a wrench. An emphatic message often comes from those in mourning who are given the infuriating, well-meant advice, 'You must be strong.' A recently bereaved friend told us just how hard this was for her to hear. She had been strong and resilient all through her husband's illness. Her faith gave her inner strength to cope from day to day as her partner became weaker. Her friends and family sturdily supported them both. Hearing that phrase, she was angry that everyone's strength through the dying days was not acknowledged – but more than that: people have to be able to let go and simply mourn. Grieving well is not always 'being strong'.

Grieving is a process. Perhaps it is better just to be open to grief from day to day as the healing process begins. There will be days of light and peace, and others when the build-up of tension and exhaustion overwhelm you and the thought of getting out of bed is just too daunting. Give in to the body's desire to rest and sleep. Seek help if this becomes a daily problem.

It takes at least eighteen months to two or three years, depending on the circumstances, for life to return to normal. Suddenly you wake up one morning and realise that 'that pain in the solar plexus' – that dull ache – and bouts of tearfulness have diminished. You find you can say the name of your beloved more easily. You will notice that you do not feel devastated and conflicted with this. The sun shines as brightly as it used to, the rain and wind refresh the earth, and the scent of jasmine smells just as it should.

# Appendix:
# Texts for reflection

The tragedy of life is not in the fact of death. The tragedy of life is what dies inside a man while he lives – the death of genuine feeling, the death of inspired response; the death of awareness that makes it possible to feel the pain or the glory of other men in oneself . . . No man need fear death: he need fear only that he may die without having known his greatest power – the power of his free will to give his life for others.

*Albert Schweitzer*


I feel and know that death is not the ending, as we thought, but rather the real beginning – and that nothing ever is or can be lost, nor even die, nor soul, nor matter.

*Walt Whitman*

Death is a dialogue between
The spirit and the dust.
'Dissolve,' says Death. The Spirit, 'Sir,
I have another Trust.'

Death doubts it, argues from the ground.
The Spirit turns away,
Just laying off, for evidence,
An overcoat of clay.

*Emily Dickinson*

Our life essence, our connection to meaning, truth,
and beauty, our deep relationship to self and others is all
part of spirituality. To love and be loved, to be respected; to be forgiven. To be validated, to be understood.
These are all crucial spiritual needs. Death offers us a
chance to see the spiritual wherever we look. To see the
sacred in simple objects.

*Peter Fox*

That which dies in a man is only his five senses. That
which continues to exist, beyond his senses, is immense,
unimaginable, sublime.

*Anton Chekov*

When death comes
like the hungry bear in autumn;
when death comes and takes all the bright coins
from his purse

to buy me, and snaps the purse shut;
when death comes
like the measle-pox:

when death comes
like an iceberg between the shoulder blades,

I want to step through the door full of curiosity,
wondering
what is it going to be like, that cottage of darkness?

When it's over, I don't want to wonder
if I have made my life something particular, and real.
I don't want to find myself sighing and frightened,
or full of argument.
I don't want to end up simply having visited this world.

*Mary Oliver*

How do the geese know when to fly to the sun? Who tells them the seasons? How do we, humans, know when it is time to move on? As with the migrant birds, so surely with us, there is a voice within, if only we would listen to it, that tells us so certainly when to go forth into the unknown.

*Elisabeth Kübler-Ross*


In the sweat of your face you shall eat bread till you return to the ground, for out of it you were taken; you are dust, and to dust you shall return.

*Holy Bible, Genesis 3: 19*


For everything there is a season, and a time for
every matter under heaven:
a time to be born and a time to die; a time to plant,
and a time to pluck up what is planted;
a time to kill, and a time to heal; a time to break
down, and a time to build up;
a time to weep, and a time to laugh; a time to
mourn, and a time to dance;
a time to cast away stones, and a time to gather
stones together;
a time to embrace, and a time to refrain from
embracing;

a time to seek, and a time to lose; a time to keep,
and a time to cast away,
a time to rend, and a time to sew; a time to keep
silence, and a time to speak;
a time to love, and a time to hate; a time for war,
and a time for peace.

*Holy Bible, Ecclesiastes 3: 1–9*


What can we know of death, we who cannot
understand life?
We study the seed and the cell, but the power deep
within them will always elude us.
Though we cannot understand, we accept life as the
gift of God. Yet death, life's twin, we face with fear.
But why be afraid? Death is a haven to the weary,
a relief for the sorely afflicted. We are safe in death
as in life.
There is no pain in death. There is only the pain of
the living as they recall shared loves, and as they
themselves fear to die.
Calm us, O Lord, when we cry out in our fear and
in our grief. Turn us anew toward life and the world.
Awaken us to the warmth of human love that speaks
to us of You.
We shall fear no evil as we affirm Your kingdom of life.

*From Gates of Prayer: The New Union Prayer Book*

[The Lord] said to me 'My grace is sufficient for you,
for my power is made perfect in weakness.'
I will all the more gladly boast of my weakness,
that the power of Christ may rest upon me.

*Holy Bible, 2 Corinthians 12: 9–10*


Since therefore the children share in flesh and blood,
he himself likewise partook of the same nature,
that through death he might destroy him who has
the power of death, that is, the devil,
and deliver all those who through fear of death were
subject to lifelong bondage.

*Holy Bible, Hebrews 2: 14–15*


O Lord, support us all the day long of this troublous
life, until the shades lengthen, and the evening comes,
and the busy world is hushed, the fever of life is over,
and our work is done.
Then, Lord, in your mercy grant us safe lodging, a holy
rest, and peace at last; through Jesus Christ our Lord.

*From the funeral service,*
*Church of the Province of South Africa*

Deep peace of the running wave
to you.
Deep peace of the flowing air
to you.
Deep peace of the quiet earth
to you.
Deep peace of the shining stars
to you.
Deep peace of the infinite peace
to you.

*Adapted from Gaelic runes*


Look to this day! For it is life. The very life of life.
For yesterday is only a dream, and tomorrow
    is only a vision.
But today, well lived, makes every yesterday a dream
of happiness and every tomorrow a vision of hope.

*The Holy Quran*


Our Lord! Pour out on us patience and constancy,
and make us die as those who have surrendered
themselves unto You.

*The Holy Quran 7: 126*

Be sure we shall test you
With something of fear
And hunger, some loss
In goods or lives or the fruits
Of your toil, but give glad tidings to those
Who patiently persevere,
Who say, when afflicted
With calamity: 'To God we belong,
And to Him is our return.'
They are those on whom
(descend) blessings from God,
And mercy,
And they are the ones
That receive guidance.

*The Holy Quran 11: 155–157*


Not teach ripe person! Waste of person.
Teach not ripe person! Waste of words.

*Confucius*

Wisdom is the finest beauty of a person.
Money does not prevent you from becoming blind.
Money does not prevent you from becoming mad.
Money does not prevent you from becoming lame.
You may be ill in any part of your body, so it is
Better for you to go and think again
And to select wisdom,
Come and sacrifice, that you may rest in your
Body,
Inside and outside.

*Traditional African prayer*


Let us behave gently,
that we may die peacefully;
That our children may stretch out their hands
Upon us in burial.

*Prayer from Yoruba, Nigeria*

# Useful contacts

This information was correct as far as we could ascertain at the time of writing, in February 2005.

## AIDS

**AIDS Action Group**
021 948 7699 (Cape Town)
aag@icon.co.za

**AIDS Education Unit**
021 448 7312 (Cape Town)

**AIDS Helpline (24-hour counselling lines)**
They also offer face-to-face counselling.

| | |
|---|---|
| Countrywide | 086 132 2322 |
| Alexandra | 011 443 3555 |
| Cape Town | 021 461 1111 |
| East London | 043 722 2000 |
| East Rand | 011 422 4242 |
| Johannesburg | 011 728 1347 |

| North West Province | 086 132 2322 |
| Port Elizabeth | 041 585 5581 |
| Pretoria | 012 342 2222 |
| Soweto | 011 988 0155/6 |
| West Rand | 011 665 2281 |
| KwaZulu-Natal | 086 132 2322 |

**AIDS Legal Networks**
021 423 9254 (Cape Town)
aln@kingsley.co.za

**AIDS Training and Information and
Counselling Centre**
021 797 3327 (Cape Town)

**Anglican AIDS**
1A Braehead House, Kenilworth, Cape Town.
PO Box 53113, Kenilworth 7745
021 762 4220, fax 021 762 4237
info@anglicanaids.org
www.anglicanaids@org

**HIVAN Centre for HIV/AIDS Networking**
University of KwaZulu-Natal, Public Affairs Annexe,
232 King George V Avenue, Durban 4041
031 260 3334, fax 031 260 2013
eliazm@hivan.org.za or admin@hivan.org.za

They offer a wide selection of services and information and in particular bereavement counselling.

**Book, music and tape orders by Web**
www.amazon.com
www.exclusivebooks.com (Exclusive Books)
www.onlineshopping.co.za (South Africa Online Shopping)
www.tapeaids.co.za (Tape Aids for the Blind)
www.cdselectonline.co.za (CD Select Online)
www.musica.co.za (Musica)

**Cancer**

**Cancer Association of South Africa**
cansainfo@cansa.org.za
www.cansa.org.za

**Cancer Bacup**
www.cancerbacup.org.uk
Cancer support service

**CISS Trust (Cancer Information and Support Services Trust)**
PO Box 2881, Parklands, Johannesburg 2121
011 642 4562/3, fax 011 484 1310
cisstrust@icon.co.za

**The National Cancer Association of South Africa (CANSA)**
National office: 26 Concorde Road West, Bedfordview, Johannesburg
PO Box 2121, Bedfordview 2008
011 616 7662, fax 011 622 3424,
tollfree helpline 080 022 6622
cancerjhb@cancer.org.za
www.cansa.org.za

**The Cancer Information Service (in Cape Town)**
Tollfree 080 022 6622

Local contacts:
Cape Town: 021 689 5347, fax 021 685 1937,
  cjeffrey@eagle.mrc.ac.za
Eastern Cape: 041 373 8133
Free State and Northern Cape: 051 444 2580
Gauteng: 011 646 5628, fax 011 646 2914
Northern Province: 012 329 3036
KwaZulu-Natal: 031 205 9525

A private, non-profit, registered welfare organisation. It offers research, education and community services which include counselling, pain control and support for patients.

## Hospice

### Hospice Association of South Africa
PO Box 38785, Pinelands 7430
021 531 2094, fax 021 531 7917
For all information on Hospices nationwide,
contact the above number.

## Hospitals

### Health FAQ South Africa
www.safrica.info/public_services/citizens/health/
healthfaq2.htm
Information on public and private hospitals.

## National medical bodies

### Allied Health Professions Council of South Africa
PO Box 31565, Wonderboompoort 0033
61 Rose Street, Riviera, Pretoria 0084
012 329 4001, fax 012 329 2279
healthco@mweb.co.za
www.ahpcsa.co.za

### Alzheimer's South Africa
P O Box 81183, Parkhurst, Johannesburg 2120
011 478 2234, fax 011 478 2251
info@alzheimers.org.za
www.alzheimers.org.za

**Health Professions Council of South Africa**
553 Vermeulen Street, Arcadia, Pretoria
PO Box 205, Pretoria 0001
012 338 9300, fax 012 329 2279
ahpcsa@hspcsa.co.za

Every health professional in South Africa must
be registered with this new statutory body.

**Massage Therapy Association South Africa**
021 671 5313 (and fax)
PO Box 53320, Kenilworth, Cape Town 7745
www.mtasa.co.za

**Motor Neuron Disease Association of South Africa**
PO Box 191, Milnerton 7435
Contact: Rina Myburgh (secretary) 021 531 9744,
fax 021 531 6222 (Cape Town)
mndaofsa@global.co.za

**Multiple Sclerosis Society of South Africa**
National helpline 086 045 6772
www.multiplesclerosis.co.za

**Muscular Dystrophy Foundation of South Africa**
National office: Room 111, NRDI House,
11 Mackay Avenue, Blairgowrie, Johannesburg
national@mdsa.org.za

**Parkinsonian Association of South Africa**
P Bag X36, Bryanston 2021
011 787 8792, fax 011 787 2047
parkins@global.co.za

**South African Medical Association**
PO Box 74789, Lynwood Ridge, Pretoria 0040
Block F, Castle Walk, Corporate Park, Nossob Street,
Erasmuskloof X3, Pretoria
012 481 2000, fax 012 481 2100
www.samedical.org

**South African National Tuberculosis Association
(SANTA)**
National office: P Bag X10030, Edenvale 1610
011 454 0200, fax 011 454 0096
santa@santa.org.za
www.santa.org.za

**The South African Reflexology Society**
National chair: G Hansen 021 712 2455
Mon–Fri 8–12 am (Cape Town)
gailh@iafrica.com

Also see Reflexology Society of South Africa
under Therapies.

**Traditional Medical Practitioners of South Africa**
PO Box 4340, Johannesburg 2000
011 333 7839, fax 011 333 7674

## Miscellaneous information

### Citizens' Advice Bureau
37 Schoeman Street, Pretoria 0002
012 322 6630, fax 012 320 2114

Free information service on your rights;
a guide to other helpful services.

### Free Spirit
021 447 3600, fax 021 447 3610
abreeze@iafrica.com
www.freespiritsa.co.za

This is a weekly lifestyle magazine TV show
focusing on issues of mind, body and spirit,
created by Shoot the Breeze Productions.

### The Living Will Society (Saves)
PO Box 1460, Wandsbeck 3631, KwaZulu-Natal
031 266 8511, fax 031 267 2218
www.livingwill.co.za

**Up-U-Go hoist**
Contact: Julian Baring-Gould 021 852 1683 or
083 467 3656 or via www.multiplesclerosis.co.za

## Nursing

**St John Ambulance**
National office: cnr Leyds and Loveday streets,
Braamfontein, Johannesburg
PO Box 744, Johannesburg 2000
011 403 4227, fax 011 403 2533
www.stjohn.org.za

Contact for offices nationwide: they are in every
major centre in South Africa.
First-aid training, and basic and advanced home-care
courses.

## Personal support

**Compassionate Friends**
National chair: Richard Morris,
9 Whites Road, Waverley 9305
051 522 17130 (Bloemfontein)
www.health24.com/mind/Support_groups/

For details of the branches nationwide
or contact the Cape Town chapter:

Cynthia Lassen, 30 Belgrave Circle,
Atlantic Beach Golf Estate, Melkbosstrand 7441
021 553 0038
cyndre@telkomsa.net

Alta Swanepoel, PO Box 913, Somerset West 7129
021 856 0717
aswannie@mweb.co.za

**Depression and Anxiety Group**
PO Box 652548, Benmore 2010
011 783 1474/6, after hours 080 011 9283
anxiety@iafrica.com

**LifeLine South Africa**
National office: 10th Floor, North City House,
cnr Jorissen and Melle streets, Braamfontein,
Johannesburg 2001
PO Box 32201, Braamfontein 2017
24-hour counselling lines 011 728 1347
(Johannesburg), 021 461 1111 (Cape Town)

For contact numbers of other branches nationwide,
contact either of the above two numbers.
24-hour crisis line countrywide 086 132 2322
They also offer a face-to-face counselling service.

**Nechama (Bereavement counselling division of the Jewish Helping Hand and Burial Society)**
Johannesburg: PO Box 51531, Raedene 2124
011 640 1322
Cape Town: Pauline Sevitz, Highlands House,
9 Gorge Road, Oranjezicht, Cape Town 8001
021 465 9390

**Social welfare grants**
Department of Social Development
www.socdev.gov.za/Services/ugrant.htm

Website information: Grants available,
Applying for grants, Monetary value of grants.

**Spiritual and mental life**
The Buddhist Information Centre
6 Morgenrood Road, Kenilworth, Cape Town 7700
021 785 2676

**The Centre for Christian Spirituality**
1 Chapel Road Lane, Rosebank, Cape Town 7700
021 686 1269 (mornings only)
christianspirit@xsinet.co.za

For information on meditation and other topics:
see the monthly magazine *Odyssey*, available from
most bookstores. It has a large directory of
practitioners of all kinds.

## Therapies

### The Dr Edward Bach Centre
Mount Vernon, Bakers Lane, Sotwell, OX10 OPZ,
United Kingdom.
www.Bachcentre.com

### Body Stress Release Association of South Africa
PO Box 569, Wilderness 6560
021 7883081 (Cape Town), 044 883 1026 (Wilderness)
e-gmeg@mweb.co.za

### Massage Therapy Association South Africa (MTA)
PO Box 53320, Kenilworth 7745
021 6715313 (and fax)
www.mtasa.co.za

### The Reiki Association of South Africa
karen@reikiassociation.co.za
www.soulhealing.co.za

### The South African Reflexology Society
Contact: G Hansen 021 712 2455
Mon–Fri 8–12 am
http://www.sareflexology.org.za

### *Disclaimer*
The authors of this book, their publishers or agents do
not accept any responsibility for any claims made by
organisations, individuals or products listed above.

# References

Betts, Donni and George Betts. *Growing Together*. Millbrae, CA: Celestial Arts, 1973.

Bly, Robert, James Hillman and Michael Meade (eds). *The Rag and Bone Shop of the Heart: Poems for Men*. New York, NY: Harper Collins, 1992.

Brussat, Frederick and Mary Anne, *Spiritual Literacy: Reading the Sacred in Everyday Life*. New York, NY: Scribner, 1996.

Buckman, Robert. *I Don't Know What to Say: Communicating with Dying Patients*. London: Macmillan, 1988; New rev. ed. London: Papermac, 1990.

Cassidy, Sheila. *Sharing the Darkness: The Spirituality of Caring*. London: Darton, Longman and Todd, 1988.

Chancellor, Philip. *The Illustrated Handbook of the Bach Flower Remedies*. Saffron Walden, Essex: CW Daniel, 1980.

Chopra, Deepak. *The Seven Spiritual Laws of Success: A Practical Guide to the Fulfilment of Your Dreams*. London: Bantam/Transworld, 1996.

Cole, Roger. *Mission of Love: A Physician's Spiritual Journey Toward a Life Beyond*. Berkeley, CA: Celestial Arts, 2002.

Commin, Bob and Viv Stacey. *Someone Dreaming Us*.
Cape Town: Mercer, 1997.

Davis, Patricia. *Aromatherapy: An A–Z*. Saffron Walden, Essex:
CW Daniel; Revised edition 2004.

Davis, Patricia. *Subtle Aromatherapy*. Saffron Walden, Essex:
CW Daniel, 1991.

Doyle, Derek. *The Platform Ticket: Memories and Musing
of a Hospice Doctor*. Durham, UK: Pentland, 1999.

Frankl, Viktor E. *Man's Search for Meaning*. London: Hodder
& Stoughton, 1964.

Fynn. *Mister God This Is Anna*. London: Fountain/Collins, 1977.

Grollman, Earl A. *Living When a Loved One Has Died:
A Collection of Poetry*. Boston, Mass.: Beacon Press, 1977.

Grosz, Anton. *Letters to a Dying Friend: Helping Those You
Love Make a Conscious Transition*. Wheaton, Ill.: Quest
Books, Theosophical Publishing House, 1997.

Harrison, Gavin, *In the Lap of the Buddha*. Boston, Mass.:
Shambhala, 1994.

Gwilliam, Rob, Shea Albert, Hank Albert and Steven Albert.
*Pathways to Healing: The Story of Jessie Albert*.
Johannesburg: The Jessie Albert Resource Centre, 2000.

Kearney, Michael. *A Place of Healing: Working with Suffering
in Living and Dying*. Oxford: OUP, 2000.

Kübler-Ross, Elisabeth. *Death, the Final Stage of Growth:
On Death and Dying*. London: Routledge, 1989 (1975).

Kübler-Ross, Elisabeth. *The Tunnel and the Light*. New York,
NY: Marlowe, 1999.

Kübler-Ross, Elisabeth. *The Wheel of Life: A Memoir of Living and Dying*. New York, NY: Scribner, 1997.

Kunitz, Stanley. *Passing Through: The Later Poems*. New York, NY: WW Norton, 1995.

Lello, Sr Pat. 'Physical Aspects of Palliative Care' in *The St Luke's Hospice Training Manual*. Kenilworth, Cape Town: St Luke's Hospice, 2002.

Levine, Stephen. *Meetings at the Edge: Dialogues with the Grieving and the Dying, the Healing and the Healed*. Dublin: Gateway, 1984.

Lyall, David. *Counselling in the Pastoral and Spiritual Context*. Buckingham, UK: Open University Press, 1995.

Mayor, Ian and Deirdre Hanna. 'A Vision of Holistic Care'. Paper presented at the 13th International Congress on Care of the Terminally Ill, 25–29 September 2000, Montreal, Canada. Abstract published in *Journal of Palliative Care*, 16, 3, Autumn 2000. 63–94.

McLeod, Beth Witrogen. *Caregiving: The Spiritual Journey of Love, Loss and Renewal*. Hoboken, NJ: Wiley, 1999.

Mitchell, Stephen (ed). *The Enlightened Heart: An Anthology of Sacred Poetry*. New York, NY: Harper & Row, 1989.

Nairn, Rob. *Diamond Mind: Psychology of Meditation*. Kalk Bay, Cape Town: Kairon, 1999.

Nairn, Rob. *Living, Dreaming, Dying: Wisdom for Everyday Life from the Tibetan Book of the Dead*. Kairon Exploring Consciousness Series. Kalk Bay, Cape Town: Kairon, 2002.

Nearing, Helen (ed). *Light on Aging and Dying: Wise Words Selected by Helen Nearing*. Gardiner, Maine: Tilbury House, 1995.

Nouwen, Henri JM. *Our Greatest Gift: A Meditation on Dying and Caring*. London: Hodder & Stoughton, 1994.

Peck, M Scott. *Denial of the Soul: Spiritual and Medical Perspectives in Euthanasia and Mortality*. New York, NY: Harmony, 1997.

Sanford, D. *It Must Hurt a Lot: A Child's Book about Death*. Portland. Maine: Multnomah, 1986.

Schroeder-Sheker, Therese. 'Music for the Dying'. *Noetic Sciences Review*, 31, Autumn 1994.

Schroeder-Sheker, Therese, Paul Kaufman and Jennifer Kaufman. *Chalice of Repose: A Contemplative Musician's Approach to Death and Dying* with Therese Schroeder-Sheker. Video recording. Producer, Paul Kaufman; director, Jennifer Kaufman. Boulder, CO: Sounds True, 1997.

Siegal, Bernie S. *Love, Medicine and Miracles*. London: Arrow/Random, 1988.

Siegal, Bernie S. *Living, Loving and Healing*. London: Aquarian/Thorsons, 1993.

Staudacher, Carol. *Men and Grief: A Guide for Men Surviving the Death of a Loved One*. Place, CA: New Harbinger, 1991.

Stein, Diane. *Essential Reiki: A Complete Guide to an Ancient Healing Art*. Freedom, CA: The Crossing Press, 1995.

Stickney, Doris. *Waterbugs and Dragonflies: Explaining Death to Children*. London: Mowbray/Cassell, 1984.

Stone, Ganga. *Start the Conversation: The Book about Death You Were Hoping to Find*. New York, NY: Warner, 1996.

Tutu, Desmond. *An African Prayer Book*. London: Hodder & Stoughton, 1995.

Twycross, Robert G and Sylvia A Lack. *Oral Morphine: Information for Patients, Families and Friends*. Beaconsfield, Bucks: Beaconsfield, 1987.

Wilbur, Ken. *Grace and Grit: Spirituality and Healing in the Life and Death of Treya Killam Wilbur*. Boston, Mass.: Shambhala, 1993, 1991.

Worden, JW. *Grief Counselling and Grief Therapy*. London: Routledge, 1989.

Yancey, Philip. *What's So Amazing about Grace?* Grand Rapids, Michigan: Zondervan, 1997.

# Acknowledgements

We extend our deep gratitude to all our supporters for their generosity and enthusiasm. We greatly appreciate the help of those who spent time commenting on the draft. We learned a great deal from them. Most of all, to those who bared their very souls to us in times of vulnerability, distress, pain and joy, to help with our insights, whose names are too many to mention – thank you. Peter appreciates the support and encouragement he received from the Spiritual Care Team at St Luke's Hospice in Kenilworth.

To our editor, Priscilla Hall, our warmest thanks for bringing the whole book together with such enthusiastic professionalism. Helen Broekmann typed, corrected and improved the many transcripts with dedication. Her objective criticism and clarity have been invaluable. Thanks also go to our homeopath Dr Mary Cattell, oncologist Dr Elizabeth Murray, and chiropractor Dr Timothy Wood for valuable input, constructive criticism and time; Noel Wood for legal advice and assistance; Joan Hill, Sue's stalwart friend; Allan and Joanna Hardie for their consistent encouragement and unswerving faith in our project when we stumbled, wavered and wanted to give up; and our guardian angel, Dr Dorian Haarhoff, who graced our work with talent and imagination, bringing life to our sometimes awkward words.

We and our publishers gratefully acknowledge permission from these sources to quote from their publications:

Faber & Faber for the quotation from Dag Hammarskjöld, *Markings*, transl. Lief Sjoberg and WH Auden (1964), on p v

Beverley Rycroft for material on pp 1, 61–2

Viv Stacey for the epigraph on p 47 from *Someone Dreaming Us* by Bob Commin and Viv Stacey (1997)

Patrick van Blerk for his song 'Paradise Road' quoted on p 58

Tim Wood for his poem 'Squeezing Life's Summer' (p 64) and for information used on pp 142ff

Celestial Arts for the epigraph on p 74 from Donni and George Betts, *Growing Together* (1973)

The Hospice of Lancaster County, Pennsylvania, USA, for 'A Caregiver's Litany' by Camilla Hewson Flintermann (p 78–9) and Nine tips for carers (pp 80–1)

Harper & Row for the poem by Li Po ( p 80) in *The Enlightened Heart: An Anthology of Sacred Poetry*, ed. Stephen Mitchell (1989)

WW Norton for the poem 'Touch Me' (p 82) from Stanley Kunitz, *Passing Through: The Later Poems* (1995)

Harper Collins for the poem 'Portrait' by Antonio Machado
(p 96) in *The Rag and Bone Shop of the Heart: Poems for
Men*, ed. Robert Bly, James Hillman and Michael Meade
(1992)

JP Tarcher for the epigraph on p 97 from Sam Keen and
Anne Valley Fox, *Your Mythic Journey* (1989)

Epigraph on p 97 from www.bread4thehead.com

Robert G Twycross and Sylvia A Lack for the epigraph on
p 128 from *Oral Morphine: Information for Patients,
Families and Friends* (1987) and for material quoted on
pp 130–1

Sr Pat Lello for her 'Physical Aspects of Palliative Care' in the
*St Luke's Hospice Training Manual*, on which we drew for
ideas in chapter 12

Cynthia Birrer for the quote on pp 132–3 from 'Wages of
Love: The Experience of Loss'

The Hospice of Lancaster County, Pennsylvania, and the
Ohio Hospice and Palliative Care Organization, Ohio, for
'The Last 48 Hours: Signs and Symptoms of Approaching
Death' (pp 150–3), from which the epigraph by Dame
Cecily Saunders (p 150) comes

Beacon Press for the poem 'When Death Comes' on (p 165)
by Mary Oliver in *New and Selected Poems* (1992)

Scribner for the quotation on p 166 from Elisabeth Kübler-
Ross, *The Wheel of Life: A Memoir of Living and Dying*
(1997)

Prayer on p 167 from *Gates of Prayer: The New Union Prayer*

*Book* (London: Union of Liberal and Progressive Synagogues, 1975)

Prayer on p 168 from the Funeral Service of the Church of the Province of Southern Africa, Alternative Series 3

Benediction on p 169 from John O'Donoghue, *Eternal Echoes* (New York: Harper Collins, 1999)

Prayers on p 171 from Desmond Tutu, *An African Prayer Book* (Cape Town: Double Storey Books, 2004)

The authors and publishers have made every effort to contact the copyright holders of material quoted in this book. Should there be any omission of acknowledgement, we shall gladly rectify this in future impressions.

# About the authors

Sue Wood trained and worked as a nurse and has practised as an aromatherapist since 1982. This experience has enabled her to understand the importance of hands-on care and compassion. It has also taught her the way the body works with unexpressed fears and unprocessed emotions. Her work as a holistic aromatherapist and counsellor for the past twenty years has entailed extensive interaction with many terminally ill patients.

After an Honours degree at Rhodes University in 1973, and through 22 years of pastoral ministry in the Uniting Presbyterian Church in Southern Africa, Peter Fox has always had counselling as a special focus of interest and expertise in his vocation. He assisted in the formation of LifeLine in Port Elizabeth in 1977. Since 1996 he has been working as spiritual counsellor at St Luke's Hospice in Kenilworth, Cape Town. He lectures in the field of grief and loss and has since June 2004 been in part-time private practice. Skills of spiritual companioning and a working knowledge of psychodynamic theory influence his work.